KEY COMPETENCIES
IN BRIEF DYNAMIC PSYCHOTHERAPY

Key Competencies in Brief Dynamic Psychotherapy
Clinical Practice Beyond the Manual

JEFFREY L. BINDER

THE GUILFORD PRESS
New York   London

© 2004 The Guilford Press
A Division of Guilford Publications, Inc.
72 Spring Street, New York, NY 10012
www.guilford.com

Printed in the United States of America

This book is printed on acid-free paper.

Last digit is print number: 9 8 7 6 5 4 3 2 1

Library of Congress Cataloging-in-Publication Data

Binder, Jeffrey L.
  Key competencies in brief dynamic psychotherapy: clinical practice beyond the
manual / Jeffrey L. Binder.
      p. cm.
  Includes bibliographical references and index.
  ISBN 1-59385-058-1
  1. Psychodynamic psychotherapy.   2. Brief psychotherapy.   3. Core competencies.
  I. Title.
  RC489.P72B54 2004
  616.89′14—dc22

                                                            2004008856

To Kasey and Emily, who inspire me

To Hans

and

In memory of Marty Mayman

About the Author

Jeffrey L. Binder, PhD, ABPP, is Professor and Department Head of the Clinical Psychology Program at the Georgia School of Professional Psychology of Argosy University, Atlanta. Previously, Dr. Binder was Research Associate Professor of Psychology and Clinical Assistant Professor of Psychiatry at Vanderbilt University, Nashville, Tennessee. He was also Clinical Assistant Professor of Psychiatry at the University of Virginia, Charlottesville, and Assistant Professor of Psychiatry at the University of Michigan, Ann Arbor. Dr. Binder was the director of an outpatient community mental health clinic, and helped to develop a private psychiatric hospital, where he held various clinical administrative positions. He has also had a private practice in psychotherapy. Dr. Binder became involved in the brief psychotherapy movement during the early 1970s while on the faculty at the University of Michigan, and has been actively involved in practicing and teaching brief psychotherapy since that time. He also spent a decade involved in psychotherapy research. For the past 30 years, Dr. Binder has presented and published extensively on the topics of brief psychotherapy and psychotherapy training. The book that he coauthored with Hans H. Strupp, *Psychotherapy in a New Key: A Guide to Time-Limited Dynamic Psychotherapy*, is a classic in the area of brief dynamic treatment.

Preface

Books about psychodynamically oriented psychotherapies tend to focus on relatively broad and abstract intrapsychic forces, relationship vicissitudes, and therapeutic strategies. They present epic psychological and interpersonal events from a distance, without a detailed view of moment-to-moment transactions among the participants. Readers of the psychodynamic literature—by Freud through contemporary authors—may be captivated by the highly literate writing styles characteristically used to depict psychological forces as well as intrapsychic and interpersonal events, but just as often they are left unsure about how to recreate comparable experiences in their own therapies. Perhaps the biggest problem faced by psychodynamic authors when trying to describe how to conduct therapy is the strained attempt to utilize clinical theories and languages in efforts to depict the mental processes of therapists while they are engaged in clinical work. These clinical theories and languages were not developed to explain the complex performances of professional experts in any domain, including clinical work. This problem is especially acute in the literature on brief psychodynamic therapy, which, with few exceptions, has long been characterized by clinical theories of personality and therapy that lag behind the most contemporary theoretical and technical developments in the field. Consequently, even though many books on brief dynamic therapy reflect high levels of scholarship and clinical wisdom, they tend to be written in even more theoretically abstract and vague language than many contemporary books on long-term psychoanalytic therapy and psychoanalysis.[1]

I first became aware of the challenge of adequately depicting the mental processes and behaviors associated with competent therapist performance while participating in an extended empirical study of the impact of systematic training in brief dynamic psychotherapy on the performance of experienced therapists (Strupp, 1993). Some of the members of the research team began to look outside of the psychodynamic clinical literature for a better way to conceptualize and discuss complex performances (of which the conduct of psychotherapy certainly is an example). I became intrigued with an area of theory and research in the cognitive sciences that addresses the nature of generic expertise and the development from novice to expert across performance domains. With one exception (Schon, 1983), cognitive scientists engaged in this research have not addressed therapist performance. However, studying the investigations of other complex performance domains has provided invaluable guidance in my attempts to describe the mental processes and subjective experiences of therapists trying to conduct competent, brief dynamic–interpersonal psychotherapy.

An observation about a cardinal characteristic of the best of world-class athletes appeared in an article in *USA Today*: "The greatest players in any sport have the ability to slow things down so that they can see it, compute it and deal with it, while it's still speeding for everyone else." In baseball, for example, a great hitter is able to slow down the pitched ball, in his mind, so that he can see it better. The article quoted a typical comment from expert hitters: "When you're hitting well, it's like slow motion. You see everything." The article listed another cardinal characteristic of expert hitters as the ability to pick up subtle cues in the immediate situation, anticipate what will happen next, and quickly react. For example, Hank Aaron, the retired Atlanta Braves outfielder who holds the record for most career home runs, was quoted as saying: "When I got into a groove, it wouldn't make any difference who was out there pitching. I could always guess, and guess right" (*USA Today*, July 5, 1999, Section 3C).

Comparable observations can be made about experts in any complex performance domain, including the conduct of psychotherapy (Ericsson & Charness, 1999). When a proficient therapist is "on his or her game" or "in a groove," he or she sees and responds in a way that allows anticipation and adjustments to shape and refine the therapy session—skills unavailable when a therapist is performing merely competently. The origins and nature of interpersonal patterns are more likely to be identified, because the expert therapist draws on previous experiences in similar situations to anticipate likely patterns of behavior.[2]

The expert therapist also views interpersonal patterns with relatively more clarity because he or she sees the patterns slowly superimposing over one another, even while he or she is following the immediate unfolding of the therapy session. This form of understanding allows the therapist to make trenchant observations about regularities in interpersonal relating that pervasively influence the patient's life. The detection of these regularities can be profoundly meaningful to the patient. This incisive understanding also makes the therapist capable of implementing deft adjustments to the continually changing nuances of interpersonal interactions. He or she displays technical and interpersonal flexibility and creativity and can improvise to meet immediate therapeutic exigencies. In a study of "master therapists" conducting manualized treatments, Goldfried and his colleagues observed that these experts did not go "by the book" as much as nonexpert therapists, even if the master therapists had written the manuals (Goldfried, Raue, & Castonguay, 1998). The expert therapist "finds the groove" more frequently than those less proficient, but all therapists should strive to attain this level of competence as often as possible.

As I discuss in Chapter 1, the use of treatment manuals and specific protocols does not ensure even minimal therapeutic competence. Psychotherapy process and outcome research over the past two decades has revealed that adherence to technical rules does not assure overall therapeutic skill or even narrow technical skill (except in the strictest sense of using the prescribed techniques; Beutler & Harwood, 2000). On the other hand, an accumulating body of evidence reports that, regardless of the techniques used, a better predictor of treatment outcome is the therapist's level of skill in using the techniques (Barber, Crits-Christoph, & Luborsky, 1996).

Technical competence requires a core of fundamental knowledge about personality functioning and therapeutic change processes, as well as skills for implementing strategies to facilitate those change processes. Extensive practice in implementing clinical knowledge and skills leads to progressive proceduralization whereby implementation becomes increasingly automatized. This process, in turn, fosters increments in flexibility and creativity that facilitate effective improvisation. The competent therapist develops into a proficient therapist.

In the past few years, some manual authors have at least tacitly come to appreciate this learning process. They realize that an effective psychotherapy manual should capitalize on the therapist's use of "intuitive judgment" and plan interventions that are less slavishly mired in "evidence-based" technical protocols and more informed by an understanding of the basic principles and strategies of therapeutic change (Beutler & Harwood, 2000; Piper, Joyce, McCallum, Azim, & Ogrodniczuk, 2002; Safran & Muran, 2000).

This point of view is represented here, although there is a note-worthy difference from other recent treatment manuals. Like all treatment manuals, the therapy approach presented in this book represents a particular theory of psychotherapy. Here, the approach is broadly dynamic–interpersonal. The core principle in this theoretical approach is that internal personality structures and interpersonal patterns of relating are inextricably interrelated. In addition, however, I rely on principles and strategies derived from research in the cognitive sciences on the development of competence in various domains of complex performance. Earlier I discussed the application of this area of the cognitive sciences to the study of therapist performance. I also believe that it can inform our understanding of healthy behavior.

A fundamental component of psychological health is competence in managing interpersonal relationships. This competence requires a special set of skills. Accordingly, positive psychological change results from promoting certain generic skills in the patient, the application of which are necessary if he or she is to successfully manage interpersonal relationships. By "generic" skills, I mean those skills identified by cognitive scientists as basic to all kinds of complex performances. These skills include, for example, pattern recognition and various self-monitoring abilities.

The same generic skills that underlie a patient's ability to more successfully manage relationships also underlie a therapist's ability to competently conduct psychotherapy—which is, after all, a specialized form of relationship management. These generic skills, in turn, serve as the foundation for several higher-order "competencies" that therapists must master, regardless of theoretical orientation, in order to conduct time-limited psychotherapy successfully. In this book, I discuss each of these therapist competencies and the generic skills of which they are composed. Drawing on the cognitive science literature on the process of development from novice to expert across a variety of performance domains, a guiding presumption is that the learning experiences required to develop therapist competencies are not that much different from the learning experiences required for a psychotherapy patient to improve his or her relationship skills and, therefore, his or her quality of life.

This book can be used by psychotherapy training programs as a guide to teaching the basic competencies required to conduct dynamic–interpersonal psychotherapy, particularly the time-limited variety; it is not a treatment manual that will lead you step by step through a set of therapeutic techniques. Basic therapeutic principles, particularly those regarding therapeutic change processes, and corollary technical strategies are elucidated with as little technical jargon as possible, and as close to the subjective experience of the practicing therapist as I could capture it. The book also may prove useful for experienced practitioners, by organizing and making explicit mental processes and technical actions that many may already be using in inchoate or tacit forms.

ACKNOWLEDGMENTS

I wish to thank Kathryn Moore, Executive Editor at The Guilford Press, for encouraging me to write this book and for her helpful ideas about the early drafts. I also want to thank Jim Nageotte, Senior Editor at Guilford, for his tactful nudging to complete the book and for his contributions to improving the later drafts. Thanks in addition to Margaret Ryan for greatly improving the manuscript through her excellent copy editing. Finally, I wish to express my gratitude to the patients and therapists whose efforts taught me so much about psychotherapy and about life.

NOTES

1. Three notable exceptions are the books by Levenson (1995), Safran and Muran (2000), and Strupp and Binder (1984).
2. Cognitive scientists refer to the strategy of efficiently comprehending an immediate situation by finding parallels with previously managed situations as "analogic reasoning" (Sternberg, 1977).

Contents

1

The Key to Good Psychotherapy

There always has been a large gap between the way competent psychodynamic therapists conduct therapy in their real world practices and the way their conduct is formally depicted in the professional literature and at professional meetings. This gap was empirically demonstrated in the two-decade-long Menninger Foundation Psychotherapy Research Project (Wallerstein, 1989) and across theoretical models (Goldfried et al., 1998). What is most neglected in the formal conceptualizations of therapists' activities is their crucial reliance on common sense about living a satisfying and meaningful life, particularly in terms of interpersonal relationships. For competent and expert therapists, this common sense is refined over the years, through a multitude of personal and professional experiences. Another neglected characteristic of the conduct of good therapists is their technical flexibility—that is, their ability to respond constructively to the circumstances they face at the moment. A final essential characteristic of the competent therapist, often neglected in formal discussions, is good interpersonal skills; fortunately, this characteristic is receiving more appropriate acknowledged, at least by some (Norcross, 2002). The most promising students in graduate therapy training programs arrive with a foundation comprised of these characteristics. All too often, however, our training methods then bury this foundation under a pile of knowledge about personality, psychopathology, and rules about how to conduct therapy that are either too vague to provide useful guidance or too rigid. For extended periods of time students are completely preoccupied by the theories and facts they are expected to learn.

Therapists who turn out to be competent or expert manage to develop a way of doing therapy, to some extent, *in spite of* their training. They recover their buried common sense and flexibility, which allows them to use their inherent interpersonal skills. At that point these characteristics have been refined by the acquisition of extensive clinical knowledge and accumulating clinical experience. Unfortunately, not all therapists move in this direction. They either lacked the characteristics or, for whatever reasons, have been unable to recover them, at least in the practice of psychotherapy.

The purpose of this book is to reduce the extent to which these essential characteristics get buried during training and to accelerate their recovery, when needed. It aims to accomplish these goals by reducing the gap between the way competent therapists actually think and act while they are conducting psychotherapy and the way their thoughts and actions are formally depicted. For students who already have learned basic psychodynamic therapy concepts and principles, this book is meant to serve as a guide on how to apply these concepts and principles practically and in a time-limited format. Practicing therapists may find this book to be a useful aid in fully recovering and using their common sense, technical flexibility, and interpersonal skills in their practice of therapy.

This depiction of how to conduct psychotherapy is based on over 30 years of psychotherapy practice and training and over 20 years of involvement in treatment and training research. The clinical theory used as a conceptual framework for discussing treatment is an integration of psychodynamic–interpersonal and cognitive aspects (discussed in Chapter 2). The treatment model also represents what has been called "assimilative integration" (Lazarus & Messer, 1991; Messer, 1992), which refers to reliance on a predominant theoretical framework, within which principles and techniques from other treatment models are incorporated.

My strategy for minimizing the gap between how good therapists actually think and act and how I depict their performances is to avoid, or at least minimize, the use of clinical language to describe therapist performances. Although useful for dealing with clinical issues, the languages of clinical theories are ill suited for the job of adequately depicting the mental processes and actions associated with a complex skillful performance, such as that of conducting psychotherapy (Binder, 1993, 1999). As a more effective alternative, I rely on a theoretical framework and language from the cognitive sciences, as noted in the Preface. I employ a conceptual framework for understanding the generic skills that appear to underlie all domain-specific performances (Chi, Glaser, & Farr, 1988; Feltovich, Ford, & Hoffman, 1997; Schon, 1983). My approach is to focus on generic skills that appear to underlie and support the effective implementation of techniques associated with clinical theories and theory-guided models of treatment, particularly those of a dynamic–interpersonal model. Most people have acquired these generic skills, to some degree, because they are required for successfully managing the challenges of living, including managing interpersonal relations. These skills include recognizing recurrent interpersonal patterns, the disciplined use of curiosity, common sense, and self-reflection. The process of learning theory-guided therapy principles and techniques *should* allow trainees to preserve their relevant generic skills and facilitate the use of these skills to guide the implementation of techniques.

With sufficient practice, the novice therapist can develop into a practitioner who can implement treatment models in a competent manner. Master therapists, in contrast, are capable of transcending the technical parameters dictated by treatment models. They are able to *improvise*, which means they are able to further therapeutic progress by whatever creative means necessary, given the circumstances—which are often unforeseen. The ability to improvise is one of the essential features that characterizes experts, be they psychotherapists, physicians, professional actors, musicians, professional athletes, or representatives of any other performance domain. Throughout this book, I maintain a focus on what I consider to be therapeutically relevant generic skills as well as the general clinical skills derived from them. Mastery of these generic and general clinical skills is required to become a competent, and eventually an expert, therapist.

ASSUMPTIONS ABOUT EMPIRICALLY SUPPORTED TREATMENTS AND TREATMENT MANUALS

The idea that the foundation of competent and expert psychotherapy practice consists of the flexible deployment of various skills, culminating in technical improvisation, diverges from the view prevalent among health care policymakers. The pressure to reduce health care costs has motivated the various stakeholders in the health care system to develop strategies for delivering care more efficiently and, hopefully, effectively. The prevalent view is that efficiency can be maximized, as well as effectiveness, by precisely determining the disorder or problem and addressing it with a treatment or technical protocol that has been empirically found to resolve the disorder or problem with maximum efficiency and effectiveness.[1] This view is most vigorously promoted by managed care organizations, which can increase their profits by reducing the expenditure of health care funds. Consequently, these organizations are constantly seeking practice guidelines that will increase at least the efficiency of health care treatments. The medical field has responded with various sorts of "evidenced-based" practice guidelines. In the mental health field, the American Psychiatric Association responded with treatment guidelines for several disorders and mental illnesses (e.g., unipolar depression, bipolar disorder, eating disorders, substance abuse (American Psychiatric Association, 1994). Organized psychology, through the American Psychological Association, responded to the psychiatrists' actions with its own Division 12 Task Force on the Promotion and Dissemination of Psychological Procedures, which published—and continues to publish—a growing list of approved psychotherapeutic treatments for specifically designated categories of "disorders" (Chambless & Ollendick, 2001). These "empirically supported" treatments have produced positive outcomes under controlled research conditions across several studies and therefore are considered superior to treatments that have not been put to this kind of test.

Those who put their faith in the effectiveness of empirically supported therapies also tend to put their faith in the use of treatment manuals as the foundation for training therapists in the use of effective treatment methods. Treatment manuals were originally developed by psychotherapy research teams for the purpose of improving the internal validity of research studies by precisely explicating the technical principles, strategies, and tactics of a therapy model (e.g., Barlow & Cerny, 1988; Beck, Rush, Shaw, & Emery, 1979; Klerman, Weissman, Rounsaville, & Chevron, 1984; Luborsky, 1984; Strupp & Binder, 1984). Although these manuals usually originate as part of research protocols, increasingly they are being used as all-purpose texts for students and more experienced practitioners. In fact, their use is being promoted as a requirement for accreditation of clinical psychology training programs (Crits-Christoph, Frank, Chambless, Brody, & Karp, 1995). Treatment manuals have contributed to the formulation of a more precise language for describing and explaining technical strategies and interventions, and they are associated with increased therapist adherence to the techniques prescribed in the models being taught (Binder, 1993).

The use of treatment manuals as an innovative method for enhancing psychotherapy training was greeted with tremendous optimism (Luborsky & De Rubeis, 1984; Strupp, Butler, & Rosser, 1988). Evidence does indicate that manuals are useful training tools for decreasing variance attributed to therapists in controlled studies—which was, after all, their original intent (Crits-Christoph & Mintz, 1991). After two decades of experience in using manuals in controlled studies of therapy process and outcome, however, this training innovation has not resulted in the large increment in therapist competence or effectiveness that was anticipated (Addis, 1997; Henry, Schacht, Strupp, Butler, & Binder, 1993; Lambert & Bergin, 1994; Miller & Binder, 2002). Treatment manuals usually are designed to guide the therapy of specific, circumscribed problems by applying specific techniques. A controlled research context oversimplifies the complexity and ambiguity of clinical problems encountered in actual practice. Therefore, if manuals have not made a significant impact on therapists' performances in controlled research settings, it is highly unlikely they will have a noticeable impact on real-world practitioners. Indeed, a decade after publishing his optimistic view of the potential of treatment manuals to enhance therapy research and training, Strupp (Strupp & Anderson, 1997) expressed concern about the "blind acceptance" of manuals as an effective means of improving therapist performance.

The fundamental presumption in the promotion of empirically supported treatments is that correctly chosen technical interventions are the primary determinant of therapeutic change and positive treatment outcome. Furthermore, treatment manuals are the best method of disseminating information about these correct techniques. Nevertheless, over two decades of manual-guided psychotherapy process and outcome research "have not produced support for more superior treatments or sets of techniques for specific disorders" (Lambert & Ogles, 2004, p. 167). Furthermore, "little evidence exists that efficacious treatments are readily transportable [from controlled research conditions to real-world practice]. Similarly, little evidence supports the notion that specific techniques make a substantial contribution to treatment effects" (Lambert & Ogles, 2004, p. 176).

Although there may be a host of reasons for these findings, I want to focus on two. First, practitioners working in real-world contexts are unlikely to limit themselves to specific treatment protocols designed for isolated disorders, because most patients desire help for a mix of symptomatic, interpersonal, and environmental difficulties that defies the circumscribed diagnoses used to generate outcome criteria in controlled studies. Second, even in controlled treatment trials, where there is an attempt to standardize therapists' performances, there remains significant variability in competence and effectiveness across therapists and across patients for any given therapist (Beutler, 1997; Blatt, Sanislow, Zuroff, & Pilkonis, 1996; Garfield, 1997; Lambert & Okiishi, 1997, 1986). Luborsky and his colleagues (Luborsky, McClellan, Diguer, Woody, & Seligman, 1997) used an innovative research strategy that involved compiling data from sufficient numbers of therapists who have treated sufficient numbers of patients in research studies in order to use each therapist's caseload as the unit of measure. Accordingly, therapists' caseloads could be compared for relative treatment effectiveness. Significant differences in therapeutic effectiveness across therapists again were demonstrated, with some therapists identified as generally ineffective and others as generally effective. Even the most effective therapists, however, demonstrate noteworthy variability in effectiveness across patients, although they tended to be relatively more effective with difficult patients than were the less effective therapists (Najavits & Strupp, 1994). In sum, the argument can be made that what needs to be identified are not empirically supported treatments but empirically supported *psychotherapists* (Lambert & Ogles, 2004).

Regardless of the evidence, those who have advocated for the use of treatment manuals and empirically supported treatments have achieved a hegemony in public policy. How has this development come to pass? The turmoil around health care financing is one exacerbating factor. A more fundamental and enduring reason, however, is that the advocates embody a positivistic epistemology of clinical practice (both in the mental health and general medical fields) that has attained supreme influence with health care administrators—with the support of many researchers, educators, and practitioners. This philosophy of practice posits that "standards of care" associated with specific technical strategies and interventions should be developed for each disorder. These standards of care should be derived from the findings of treatment outcome research. It is presumed that deviations from these standards would produce inefficient and ineffective treatment (Elstein, 1997). Accordingly, the core of a training program should be a treatment manual and the program's primary aim should be students' consistent adherence to empirically supported techniques.

In the health sciences the striving to develop standards of quality care is salutary, as is the desire to use empirical evidence to guide development of these standards. Unfortunately, in the mental health field such efforts are often associated with the tacit attitude that psychotherapy involves no more than a dispensing or delivery of the proper set of techniques and can be accomplished by anyone following the right format. Accordingly, it has been reported that "most managed care companies . . . regard doctoral-level practitioners as overtrained and overqualified to spend most of their time performing psychotherapy" (Cummings & Sayama, 1995, p. 29). One position held by some mental health teachers/researchers is that psychotherapies that have been used in clinical trails "have been standardized and manualized, enabling any reasonably intelligent, well-motivated 'generic therapist' to administer them" (Detrie & McDonald, 1997, p. 203). Although this approach to practice has a scientific aura, it does not have a scientific foundation, as evidenced by the research cited above. Indeed, it justifies the warning about the "uniformity myth" made by the respected psychotherapy researcher Donald Kiesler (1966) to his colleagues years ago; namely, to avoid the assumption that all therapists of a given "school" practice alike. This myth, however, also can be applied to the assumption that all therapists trained with the same manual treat their patients with equal competence.

The delivery-based view of psychotherapy is a specific case of a more general positivistic strategy that has had enormous influence on both scientific research paradigms and professional training. The social scientist Donald Schon (1983, 1987) has termed this strategy "technical rationality": The basic principle is that problem solving is made rigorous by the application of scientific theory and technique to clearly defined problems with clearly defined goals. But Schon argues that many, if not most, practice situations are not so clear-cut, whatever the professional discipline. On the contrary, many practice situations are characterized by ill-defined problems; they are "indeterminate zones" of uncertainty, instability, uniqueness, and value conflict (Schon, 1983, 1987). What an apt characterization of the typical psychotherapy session! The patient typically evidences more complex problems than are targeted in treatment efficacy studies (Seligman, 1998). Furthermore, the interaction of a particular therapist and a particular patient creates interpersonal dynamics unique to that therapeutic dyad, resulting in context-dependent technical challenges for that therapist.

Competent performance in a context such as psychotherapy— where the problems to be addressed continuously shift their form, the contextual meanings of actions continually change, and the therapist is immersed in an emotionally charged interpersonal relationship that must be effectively managed—requires more than the straightforward implementation of prescribed techniques. What *is* required are complex interpersonal skills deployed under the guidance of very sophisticated mental activities. The use of techniques associated with a particular model of treatment or with an eclectic strategy is not synonymous with competent (or expert) performance (Addis, 1997). Therapeutic techniques must be used with skill and within the containment of a positive patient–therapist relationship. Unfortunately, even clinical theorists who have recognized the multidimensional nature of therapist performance are influenced by the positivistic viewpoint, reflected in the optimistic expectation that treatment manuals eventually would evolve to a level of precision that would be sufficient to ensure skillful technical performance (Schaffer, 1982, 1983).

On the contrary, I propose that the skillful use of therapeutic techniques is ultimately based on an ability to *flexibly* adapt them to immediate contextual circumstances. All other forms of skill require this fundamental capacity. Whether choosing a surgeon for an operation or a mechanic to work on a car, the intention is to select an expert at the task, not merely someone who can "go by the book." What differentiates an "expert" from a by-the-book person? Expertise transcends simple competence to reflect the most skillful level of performance. This performance level involves the ability to deal effectively with conditions of the moment, whether routine, unique, novel, unexpected, puzzling, or critical. In other words, it is the ability to *improvise* when necessary. Going by the book—or the manual—may suffice when conditions are routine, but real skill is needed when the unexpected occurs.

IMPROVISING: THE SUPREME THERAPIST SKILL

When "master" therapists representing different treatment models conduct therapy, they tend to act more like each other than like the less skillful adherents of their own models (Goldfried et al., 1998). Indeed, the highly competent representatives of a treatment model often do not conduct therapy in the technically straightforward manner that is portrayed in the training manuals of their treatments, even when they are the authors of those manuals. For example, after viewing a videotape of Aaron Beck conducting cognitive therapy, a student of Beck's expressed surprise at the discrepancy between the official manual version of how to conduct this form of treatment and the manner in which Beck actually dealt with a difficult therapeutic situation: "Apparently, the actual practice of CT was richer in its handling of the therapeutic relationship than the textbooks would have had us believe, even then" (Newman, 1998, p. 96). A related observation from a study of cognitive and interpersonal treatments of patients with unipolar depression was that therapists who deviated from the manual-prescribed approaches in a way that made sense, particularly with difficult patients, tended to be judged as more competent (O'Malley et al., 1988). Expert therapists perform therapy in a way that distinguishes them, even from those who are using the same treatment model. The primary distinctive characteristic of these expert therapists is that they improvise, particularly in difficult situations. The necessity of improvising grows out of the inherent structure of any complex, problematic situation.

The capacity to improvise is made possible, *on the one hand*, by the acquisition and mental organization of knowledge and skills that are relevant to specific performance domains. In other words, experts improvise, but only within their specific areas of expertise. On the other hand, there are certain types of knowledge organization and basic skills that cognitive scientists have found to be associated with all of the complex performance domains that they have empirically studied. The findings from the efforts of cognitive scientists to study the development of generic expertise can be applied to better understand the mental processes and performances of psychotherapists (Binder, 1999).

Novices in any complex performance domain first acquire what is called "declarative" knowledge. This form of knowledge consists of facts, theories, principles, and rules about a knowledge domain. For example, therapy treatment manuals facilitate the understanding of abstract theories and empirically based facts about psychotherapy by rendering this type of knowledge in the form of precise technical strategies and tactics. However, whether we are playing golf, playing a musical instrument, or doing psychotherapy, a complex set of skills cannot be developed by merely reading and talking about them and observing others performing them. Simply possessing declarative theories, principles, and rules does not automatically ensure that the performer knows when and how to implement this knowledge in real-world contexts where it should guide understanding and behavior. Without additional knowledge about the appropriate and timely use of declarative knowledge, this knowledge is not spontaneously accessed when needed in the context of real-world problems. It remains "inert" (Bransford, Franks, Vye, & Sherwood, 1989). To apply the concept of inert knowledge to the work of therapy is to recognize that although a therapist may be proficient in thinking about therapy, he or she may not be proficient at actually doing therapy. Competent performers, including psychotherapists, appear to have a kind of "tacit knowing," an ostensibly ineffable sense of what to do within their performance domains (Polanyi, 1967; Sternberg & Horvath, 1999). Donald Schon (1983, 1987), a social scientist who has studied expertise in various knowledge domains, calls this tacit knowledge "knowing-in-action," to highlight the masterful performer's ability in many situations to apply his or her knowledge in spontaneous action, without deliberate thought.

Cognitive scientists refer to knowing-in-action as "procedural knowledge" and explain that this type of knowledge shapes how declarative knowledge is applied in real-world situations. In a professional context, procedural knowledge develops from the experience of applying theoretical concepts, principles, and technical prescriptions in actual psychotherapeutic contexts; it consists of the pairing of propositions and concrete experiences with action strategies and rules, as well as appraisals of the consequences. For example, when a patient complains that the therapist is unhelpful, the therapist, rather than taking it personally and becoming defensive, is immediately aware that expressions of disappointment in the therapist often reflect a transference pattern of more chronic and pervasive disappointment in others, which, if explored, often leads to therapeutic progress.

Although procedural knowledge tends to operate outside of the practitioner's conscious deliberation, it tacitly contributes to his or her "working model" of a problem context. Bowlby (1969) first developed the construct of working model to explain how humans select, organize, and store information in the process of learning to adapt to, and cope with, their environments. The working model is a kind of cognitive map that focuses on those aspects of the immediate environment relevant to the pursuit of selected goals. Although the construct was originally intended to organize explanations about general human learning, it has productively been applied to the analysis of therapist mental functioning (Peterfreund, 1983). The therapist's working model is composed of contributions from two sources. The first source is comprised of schemas. A schema is a knowledge structure that is stored in memory. It consists of conceptual information, composites of lived experiences, or a combination of both, in which discrete information is integrated into a cohesive pattern by some common theme. For example, we all have schemas that shape our views of self in various situations and interacting with specific categories of people under specific circumstances. The second source is the immediate interpersonal context (Horowitz, 1998). The therapists' working models influence (1) their use of theoretical concepts in organizing clinical information and assigning meaning to it, (2) their integration of relevant clinical data from current and past experiences, (3) their construction of coherent thematic patterns or "stories," and (4) their anticipation of events.

There is no substitute for firsthand experiences as a prerequisite for developing an intimate working knowledge of a performance domain. Competence in conducting psychotherapy is characterized by facile access to procedural knowledge that is relevant to a large variety of therapeutic situations. Procedural knowledge expands and becomes increasingly "nonconscious" and automatic with practice (Dreyfus & Dreyfus, 1988; Glaser, 1989). If not encumbered by inept performance habits, practitioners become capable of responding to a set of current practice circumstances by recalling similarly patterned experiences from previous situations as well as automatically thinking of the best strategies or actions. Competent practitioners are usually capable of acting in a reasonable and effective manner in a given the situation, without a deliberate and laborious search for the best move (Glaser, 1989; Holyoak, 1991; Kihlstrom, 1987). Relatively routine situations can be effectively managed by the partially automatized application of procedures derived from theoretical principles and professional experience. For example, in response to a patient stating that he or she does not know what to talk about, the psychodynamic therapist using the principle of "psychic determination" encourages the patient to verbalize whatever spontaneously comes to mind. The interpersonal patterns associated with such situations can be matched with prior interpersonal patterns that the therapist has encountered in a relatively straightforward manner. This matching process can be accomplished with varying degrees of conscious awareness. The therapist's current working model can be constructed with minimal effort (Cohen, Freeman, & Wolf, 1996; Schon, 1983) because his or her mental processes and behavior are guided primarily by a knowing-in-action—ability that can be only roughly described in treatment manuals.

Frequently, routine therapeutic procedural knowledge is not sufficient to deal with the vagaries of therapeutic relationships. As discussed previously, the psychotherapeutic setting is an example of a context characterized by ill-defined problems in an environment of uncertainty, instability, uniqueness, and potential value conflicts (Schon, 1983, 1987). For example, a very high percentage of people seeking psychotherapy has a mix of problems and problematic situations that makes it impossible to specify an isolated target for intervention. Furthermore, the particular characteristics that emerge within each unique patient–therapist relationship have a profound influence on the patient's assignment of meanings to the therapist's interventions—and, therefore, on the impact of these interventions.

Sometimes the most effective performance requires the capacity to switch strategies in order to make an appropriate response to a situation that contains unpredictability (Patel & Groen, 1991). This sort of adaptive flexibility is a component of the capacity to improvise as the therapeutic context continuously changes. Improvisation in any knowledge domain can be defined as the capacity to reshape understanding of the situation by reframing problems, adjusting strategies and tactics, and significantly departing from established procedures in response to novel or unexpected conditions. Because this capacity involves mental processes that occur rapidly and largely outside of awareness, it appears intuitive in nature and thus beyond the reasoning processes (Holyoak, 1991; Schon, 1983). However, improvisation appears to rely upon two identifiable sets of skills: (1) highly disciplined and automatized procedural knowledge, and (2) a highly refined self-regulatory ability that allows the person to reflect on, and adjust, his or her performance in the moment (Glaser, 1989; Schon, 1983, 1987). Whether it is a jazz musician creating an innovative riff, a golf professional shaping a difficult shot, or a cardiac surgeon performing a complex operation, improvising within the parameters of domain-relevant understandings and principles marks an expert performance.

The expert psychotherapist unwittingly has stored an enormous and largely tacit mental record of interpersonal patterns, psychological themes, therapeutic scenarios, and theoretical concepts, principles, and procedures, all organized around action–consequence sequences. Just about any interpersonal situation will activate conscious memories or at least a sense of (i.e., tacit memories) previously experienced situations or types of situations that are, to some degree, similar to the current one. These memories include previous actions that might be currently useful, and they contribute to the therapist's current working model of the therapeutic situation. As previously discussed, the activation of this sort of procedural knowledge is a tacit process. In many therapeutic situations, however, conditions are ambiguous or have potentially conflicting interpersonal meanings. Consequently, finding something familiar in the current situation is not straightforward and may even be quite difficult, because there is no obvious match with available mental records (Cohen et al., 1996; Schon, 1983, 1987). In such a predicament, the knowledge represented by these previous under-standings and actions must be reshaped to fit the unique circum-stances of the current situation. For example, the therapist senses that her patient unwittingly pushed away people with whom she would like to emotionally connect. However, the way in which the patient does this does not appear to correspond to any pattern of behavior that the therapist has seen in other patients. Nevertheless, the therapist is familiar with strategies for closely examining the patient's perceptions of her intentions that are likely to reveal the patient's unique maladap-tive actions.

This reshaping process occurs with conscious recognition, to some degree, and is the product of the other set of generic skills that under-lies expertise: the capacity for self-regulation of action. This capacity involves what cognitive scientists refer to as "metarecognition skills": knowledge of, and ability to regulate and modify, one's own mental states, processes, and behaviors (Cohen et al., 1996). The elementary form of metarecognition skill involves "reflection-on-action," either by pondering past action or by pausing in the midst of action. In the more advanced form of metarecognition skill, "reflection-in-action," delibera-tion occurs in the midst of action, without interrupting whatever is ongoing. Thinking leads to a reshaping of the performance while it is occurring (Schon, 1983, 1987). The ability to reflect-in-action requires a reshaping of the components of procedural knowledge during the pro-cess of comprehending and acting, as feedback from the situation calls for context-dependent adjustments. Self-modifications of a therapist's working model may involve revisions of the story associated with the patient's problems (in the direction of greater consistency and plausi-bility), or it may involve shifting strategies in order to overcome an ob-stacle in the patient–therapist working collaboration.

Peterfreund (1983), for example, described a "dialogue" between an operating working model and error-correcting feedback from the actual therapeutic situation. Referring to generic problem contexts, Schon (1983, 1987) described "reflective conversations" with a problem context, in which interventions reveal consequences, implications, and indicators of further actions. In the case of psychotherapy, the reflec-tive conversation is figurative, referring to the problem context, and lit-eral, referring to a collaborative dialogue with a patient. There can be two goals for such reflective conversations: (1) the construction of a therapeutically useful story to describe and explain the patient's problems, and (2) determination of the best methods for keeping the inquiry going. The most proficient form of improvisation involves reflection-in-action, whereby working models are fine-tuned or radically modified during the conduct of a therapy session through a special sort of problem-framing and problem-solving dialogue with the patient. In other words, the therapist improvises through a reflective conversation with the problem context and with the patient (Schon, 1983).

THE RELATIONSHIP BETWEEN LENGTH OF THERAPY AND OUTCOME

Therapy is most effective if it is skillfully conducted, in large part, regardless of the specific techniques used. This book focuses on how to conduct dynamic–interpersonal therapy skillfully *and* in a time-limited manner. There is no evidence to indicate how much can be accomplished in a given span of time or number of sessions if therapy is conducted with consistent competence or expertise. Over the last decade, however, solid evidence has accumulated about what can be accomplished by a very broad spectrum of therapists and patients on a very wide variety of problems, given varying amounts of time. The major innovation in research methodology that has contributed to this evidence is the "dose–effect" strategy; that is, the measurement of progressive change in therapy across treatment sessions (Howard, Kopta, Krause, & Orlinsky, 1986). The major findings regarding the individual treatment of adults are:

1. Reduction in symptoms tends to occur most quickly, whereas characterological and interpersonal problems respond more slowly to treatment.
2. Improvement tends to be greatest in the early sessions of therapy.
3. The longer the therapy, the greater the improvement, but with diminishing returns over time.
4. Across all sorts of individual therapy, 50% of patients with significant dysfunction achieve meaningful clinical improvement by the 21st session, and 75% of these patients achieve meaningful clinical improvement with at least 50 sessions.

Furthermore, treatment gains tend to endure, regardless of the length of therapy (Lambert & Ogles, 2004).[2]

The evidence is clear: On the whole, you can significantly benefit half the people you see in a traditionally defined brief treatment format (20–25 sessions), but you can substantially increase the proportion of people who benefit from your treatment if you can extend it to at least twice the length of traditionally defined brief therapies (from a traditional psychoanalytic perspective, however, a year of weekly therapy is relatively brief). It is equally clear that managed care companies that put yearly reimbursement limits on less than 50 treatment sessions are adversely affecting a substantial proportion of patients. In particular, when arbitrary limits are placed on the duration of treatment, the most likely adverse effects will be an insufficient treatment of personality patterns (affecting general as well as interpersonal functioning). Therefore, although symptom reduction may be achieved, the person may remain vulnerable to recurrence of symptoms produced by continued malfunctioning or, at least, continued malfunctioning, with the detrimental effects it has on self, others, and society. This situation is analogous to treating a bacterial infection with an arbitrary dose of medication that is insufficient to wipe out the bacteria. Symptoms may be temporarily reduced but the infection remains. Such is the logic of externally imposed treatment-session limits that are not guided by reputable research.

As the Menninger Foundation Psychotherapy Research Project revealed, long-established doctrines about the conduct, mechanisms of change, and outcomes of psychodynamic psychotherapy can be proven wrong. For example, the Menninger researchers discovered that the therapists conducting long-term expressive psychoanalytic therapy and classical analysis provided many more "supportive" interventions than would have been expected, according to theory, and the outcomes of some of the "supportive" psychotherapies indicated as much or more enduring intrapsychic "structural" change than many of the classically conducted analyses (Wallerstein, 1989). The researchers concluded that there are a variety of ways of facilitating significant psychological change.

When comparable empirical comparisons of long-term psychodynamic therapy and brief psychodynamic therapy are conducted, the same unexpected outcomes are likely to be revealed. The major differences between long-term and brief psychodynamic therapies occur in the relative impact of different change processes. In both forms of therapy, (1) cognitive insight and other forms of cognitive learning (e.g., through psychoeducation) and (2) internalized corrective interpersonal (emotional) experiences play roles in facilitating psychological change. The impact of a long-term, intimate relationship and the deep human attachment that forms between patient and therapist may result in corrective interpersonal experiences playing a relatively larger role in long-term therapy. Furthermore, because transference–countertransference enactments are much more likely to develop a prominent role in the long-term therapeutic relationship, transference interpretation is typically used more extensively. On the other hand, in the relatively shorter encounters characteristic of brief psychodynamic, interventions that promote and explicitly teach insight and interpersonal skill development may play a relatively larger role. In addition, the work may focus largely on areas of the patient's life outside therapy. These issues are discussed in more detail in Chapters 5 and 6.

In line with this perspective on the similarities and differences between long-term and brief treatments, let us consider several misconceptions about the supposedly unique technical features of brief psychodynamic therapy.

MISCONCEPTIONS ABOUT BRIEF
PSYCHODYNAMIC PSYCHOTHERAPY

Circumscribed Problem Focus and Goals

The formulation of circumscribed problems and goals is commonly cited to distinguish time-limited therapies from open-ended approaches. There is no evidence that traditional psychodynamic therapies have qualitatively different outcomes from time-limited dynamic therapies (Levenson, Butler, & Beitman, 1997), and there is strong evidence that even successful psychoanalyses do not result in complete problem resolution (Schlesinger & Robbins, 1983; Wallerstein, 1989). One implication is that problems and goals are circumscribed, to some extent, in all dynamic therapies, from psychoanalysis to time-limited dynamic treatments. Consequently, regardless of the length of treatment, the therapist should articulate a treatment focus and associated treatment goals in collaboration with the patient. The focusing process can be viewed as analogous to planning a trip with the aid of a map. Whether the ultimate destination is relatively close or far, the initial direction will be the same if both potential destinations are along the same route. The point is that there should be a planned direction for treatment regardless of its intended duration. With regard to treatment goals, when more time is available, the goals may be more ambitious but still should be specified, to some extent. In a nutshell, time-unlimited therapy is *not* characterized by an *absence* of problem definition or specified goals; that would be poorly conducted therapy. Conversely, a consistent focus on salient problems and goals is characteristic of good therapy, regardless of length.

Time Limits and Time Management

A common assumption is that time-limited therapies are, in part, defined by special attention to the management of treatment time. The setting of time limits is presumed to motivate the participants to work faster, a form of "Parkinson's Law" (Applebaum, 1975). There is as yet no solid empirical evidence to support this presumption however. Concrete arrangements for the specific length of a therapy—whether defined by number of sessions, calendar date, or by specific goals—are the relatively superficial manifestations of time management. The most expeditious management of time involves a set of attitudes about how therapeutic time should be spent and the implementation of these attitudes (Budman & Gurman, 1988; Strupp & Binder, 1984). Time should be used with maximum efficiency. In order to accomplish this objective, both therapist and patient must remain consistently focused on relevant issues, and the therapist must remain alert and actively involved in facilitating a productive working collaboration with the patient. This level of involvement should characterize a therapist's participation, regardless of the anticipated length of the treatment. Any less effort on the therapist's part would constitute inefficient work, and therefore poorly conducted therapy, regardless of the amount of time available.

Specific Selection Criteria

From Freud's epoch to the 1960s, patients' suitability for psychodynamic therapy was evaluated. In the past three decades, however, sensitivity to consumer rights has contributed to a shift in the language used with regard to treatment evaluation; the patient is now evaluated to determine if the *treatment* is suitable for him or her. Perhaps this shift was nothing more than an exercise in semantics. In any event, suitability criteria comprise some mixture of psychopathology severity and level of "ego functions"—the latter set of criteria often being unreliable because of the abstract nature of the construct. There is no empirical evidence that the vast majority of selection criteria involving patient characteristics are useful in predicting the outcome of treatment (Binder, Henry, & Strupp, 1987; Garfield, 1994). There is some evidence, however, that severity of psychopathology is a factor that can help predict rate of change (Howard et al., 1986; Kopta, Howard, Lowry, & Beutler, 1994) and that, at least in psychodynamic treatments, the effectiveness of specific therapeutic strategies is associated with the patient's maturity level of interpersonal relating (Piper, Joyce, McCallum, & Azim, 1993). Time-limited dynamic therapists have developed stringent lists of selection criteria that, essentially, include circumscribed problems, previous good adjustment, good communications skills, mature interpersonal relatedness, and high motivation (Koss & Shiang, 1994). In Chapter 3 I discuss the only patient characteristic that has shown any empirical promise as a useful predictor of the quality of therapeutic involvement; namely, the capacity for interpersonal relating. This criterion is relevant regardless of the anticipated length of treatment. In our current treatment context the primary aim of the diagnostic evaluation process is to plan intervention strategies rather than to decide whether or not treatment will be attempted. The empirical evidence has validated a suggestion made almost 20 years ago by the venerable clinician Lewis Wolberg (1980): Try all patients in time-limited therapy rather than attempting to figure out who is "suitable." Careful assessment for the purpose of treatment planning is characteristic of good therapy, regardless of length.

Therapist Activity

In the course of teaching psychotherapy and participating in process–outcome research, I have had the opportunity to listen to, or observe, the audiotaped or videotaped recordings of many therapists representing all levels of competence, in addition to reflecting on my own work. It is my conclusion that good therapists foster an active dialogue with their patients. The amount of therapist verbal activity may vary as a function of the particular type of therapy (e.g., psychoanalysis vs. brief dynamic treatment), but more likely it varies as a function of the therapist's particular work and interpersonal style. Nevertheless, the working therapeutic relationship is characterized by a dialogue rather than by a patient or therapist monologue. A competent therapist is able to deftly balance the discourse strategies of (1) facilitating candid patient communication, (2) directing the mutual exploration of the patient's salient content themes, and (3) balancing listening and intervention modes. This type of therapeutic dialogue is a hallmark of well-conducted psychotherapy, regardless of length. Furthermore, most therapist effort is directed toward the covert mental activities involved in selecting, organizing, and making sense of clinical data, in planning what to do, and appraising the nature and consequences of the unfolding therapeutic dialogue. This mental activity, conducted in a systematic, disciplined manner, is also characteristic of good psychotherapy, regardless of length.

Need to Quickly Develop a Therapeutic Alliance

A positive therapeutic alliance is the factor that psychotherapy research has shown, above all others, to be most strongly and consistently associated with positive outcome (Henry, Strupp, Schacht, & Gaston, 1994; Martin, Garske, & Davis, 2000; Orlinsky, Grawe, & Parks, 1994; Horvath & Greenberg, 1994). The expeditious establishment of a positive alliance appears to be crucial for successful treatment, regardless of length. In other words, there is no reason to conclude that unlimited treatment time reduces the need to develop and maintain a therapeutic alliance. The relatively limited time available in brief treatment leaves little opportunity for developing an alliance or fixing a broken one. The implication is that greater available treatment time offers more latitude for alliance problems. Although this argument has some merit, it does not imply that the therapist conducting open-ended therapy can passively wait for an alliance to develop without working at it, or can fix alliance problems at his or her leisure. Effective therapeutic work cannot occur without a strong alliance, so fostering the development of a therapeutic alliance should be a high priority from the inception of treatment. Similarly, dealing with alliance problems is an urgent issue in treatment of any length, if one of the goals is to maximize the efficient use of therapeutic time. Nurturing a positive therapeutic alliance is not simply a matter of being a "good person," warm, empathic, and interested. As with all intimate relationships, the therapeutic alliance takes work and is more difficult than is often presumed. The effective management of alliance issues is indicative of well-conducted psychotherapy, regardless of length.

Rapid Assessment

Strupp and Binder (1984) suggested that any distinction between evaluation and intervention efforts was artificial in practice, even if a conceptual distinction is made for teaching or research purposes. A productive therapeutic process involves, on the one hand, a therapeutic dialogue that seeks a deeper understanding of the patient throughout treatment, and, on the other hand, aims to provide some therapeutic benefit to the patient in each session. In describing the characteristics of competent problem solving across many professional domains, Schon (1987) offered this relevant aphorism: "The unique and uncertain situation comes to be understood through the attempt to change it, and changed through the attempt to understand it" (p. 132). An extension of this position is that assessment should be a high priority right from the beginning of any treatment, regardless of the anticipated length. An important component of assessment is the process of understanding the patient in order to guide and focus the type and content of interventions.

Attention to Termination Issues and Effective Management of the Process

It is commonly assumed that a distinguishing factor of time-limited therapies is the interpersonally tricky negotiation of the termination phase. Because time limits may put pressures on the patient and the therapist, it is assumed that termination will create extraordinary interpersonal stresses. Yet, the relatively brief duration of therapeutic relationships associated with time-limited treatments may, in fact, decrease the likelihood that parting will be especially difficult. The typically deeper attachments that develop in time-unlimited therapy may, on the whole, result in a greater likelihood of stress and conflict around termination. In short, there is no convincing reason or empirical evidence to presume that there are any special problems or technical strategies associated with termination issues that distinguish time-limited therapy from good psychotherapy, regardless of the length.

Therapist Optimism about What Can Be Accomplished

It has been claimed repeatedly that to be effective in using time-limited forms of therapy, the therapist must truly believe in this type of treatment (Budman & Gurman, 1988; Levenson et al., 1997). Although there is no empirical evidence to support this specific claim, common sense suggests that any effort is more likely to succeed if one has faith in the methods being used. Empirical evidence regarding the role of therapist attitudes and values in determining the fate of psychotherapy is equivocal, partly because this factor is so entwined with patient contributions to any given therapeutic dyad (Beutler, Machado, & Neufeldt, 1994). Nevertheless, those authors who advocate for systematic training in time-limited therapies often presume that once the clinician (or student) develops faith in this approach, learning how to conduct time-limited forms of therapy will be a relatively uncomplicated process. There is no empirical evidence to support this presumption. Indeed, it appears that training therapists to conduct good therapy of any length is a daunting challenge that involves guiding and shaping the development of very complex interpersonal skills.

To summarize the main implications of this section, the major consequences of time constraints are (1) that therapeutic goals may have to be circumscribed, and (2) that the therapist may explicitly have to encourage the patient to learn certain skills for managing psychological and interpersonal problems after therapy ends. These two therapeutic strategies may be relatively more important with therapies of short duration, but specifying goals (which implies some amount of circumscription) and coaching the development of certain skills are a part of any good psychotherapy. Constraints on the amount of time available for psychotherapy do not always require the therapist to work harder, to be more skillful, or to use special techniques. Good therapy is hard work for both participants, regardless of the length. Conversely, poor therapist performance will not necessarily (perhaps not usually) be compensated by the availability of more time. If a physician prescribes an ineffective type or dose of medication for some medical disorder, an unlimited duration of time for this ineffective treatment to continue does not guarantee that this error will be recognized and corrected. It is perhaps just as likely that the patient will discontinue treatment, become demoralized by medicine and physicians, or become more seriously ill. A comparable sequence of events is likely to occur with poorly conducted time-unlimited psychotherapy. It might be a very good idea to discard totally terms such as *brief, short-term,* and *time-limited* when characterizing forms of psychotherapy and replace them with terms such as *time-effective* and *time-sensitive* (Budman & Gurman, 1988). These latter terms are based on the premises that (1) most therapies are of limited duration, (2) that it is impossible to predict what goals can be achieved in a given amount of time for any given therapeutic dyad, and (3) that the secret of effective brief therapy, in regard to the therapist's role, is to conduct the treatment skillfully. I continue to use terms such as *time-limited* in this book because they are familiar, but unless stated otherwise, I am referring to the notion of *time-effective* treatment.

In sum, I do not believe that, aside from the brevity of the treatment, there is anything unique about the conduct, processes, or outcome of brief psychodynamic therapy in comparison to long-term psychodynamic therapy. *There are no specific techniques that hold the key to the practice of brief therapy. Instead, the most expeditious means to achieve efficient and effective therapeutic outcomes is to practice "good" psychotherapy, regardless of the anticipated or planned length.* In conducting brief therapy, it is especially important to identify a central issue or focus for the therapeutic work, articulate it precisely, and track it consistently within and across sessions. Conducting good psychotherapy, whether long term or brief, requires the exercise of several basic therapeutic competencies. Most of these competencies are composed of theory-guided technical strategies and tactics, although the aim of each competency is pantheoretical. In order for the therapist to improvise effectively, these competencies must be implemented with a sufficient level of skill. The competencies that I discuss were chosen partly on the basis of empirical evidence. Unfortunately, the scientific foundation of psychotherapy practice does not cover an area sufficiently wide to guide all facets of practice. It is necessary, therefore, to rely on clinical "wisdom," to some extent, which is composed, in part, of preferred theories and practices and an extensive collection of impressions and anecdotes. Drawing from these two sources of inspiration, I propose five clinical competencies that are associated with the practice of "good" dynamic–interpersonal psychotherapy.

1. *Competency in understanding personality functioning and therapeutic process.* Therapists must be able to apply (a) a clear model of personality functioning to their understanding of patients' worlds, and (b) a congruent model of therapeutic process to guide their interventions. This model of therapeutic process includes the roles of patient and therapist, how the process facilitates psychological change, and what aspects of the process may impede change. In time-limited dynamic–interpersonal psychotherapy, the process is broadly conceived of as a collaborative working relationship between patient and therapist that sometimes can be impeded by the enactment of the patient's maladaptive interpersonal patterns. These interpersonal patterns represent the expression of dysfunctional internal schemas (i.e., cognitive–affective knowledge structures) and may manifest in response to the therapist. In other words, although originating within the patient, maladaptive

interpersonal patterns may be influenced by, and in turn influence, the participation of the therapist. The enactment of interpersonal patterns that impede therapeutic change also provides a useful opportunity for understanding and acting upon the patient's problems. It is presumed that therapeutic change can be produced by several independent, or partially independent, mechanisms and processes, ranging from cognitive understanding to behavioral practice. In Chapter 2, I present models of personality functioning and therapeutic process and change that I think are a useful conceptual tools when conducting dynamic–interpersonal time-limited therapy.

2. *Competency in problem formulation and focusing.* A precise problem formulation that will serve as the focus of treatment interventions must be articulated as quickly as possible. This focus is initially incomplete and always subject to some modification and elaboration. It is a working plan of action that guides the content of the therapist's interventions. A descriptive diagnosis of psychopathology (currently represented by DSM-IV-TR categories), although ideally congruent with this formulation, is not designed to serve the same heuristic treatment function as an individually tailored formulation. In time-limited dynamic–interpersonal psychotherapy the problem formulation is conceptualized in terms of a "story" of recurrent maladaptive interpersonal patterns that reflects internal anachronistic, rigid, and dysfunctional mental working models. I discuss the assessment process and problem formulation model in Chapter 3.

3. *Competency in tracking a focus.* The problem focus serves as a guide for the content of the therapist's interventions. There is now a convincing body of empirical evidence indicating that therapist ability to track a problem focus consistently is associated with positive treatment outcome (Crits-Christoph, Cooper, & Luborsky, 1988; Messer, Tishby, & Spillman, 1992; Piper et al., 1993; Silberschatz, Fretter, & Curtis, 1986). Although there is no evidence that a precisely formulated problem focus, per se, directly contributes to a positive treatment outcome, common sense dictates that a more precisely formulated problem is easier to track. In any event, it is not known how consistently therapists can stay focused on the story content of a problem formulation, even when the precision of the formulation is enhanced by research procedures. The available evidence does not indicate that therapists do a satisfactory job of tracking a problem focus, although flaws in the research designs must be considered (Crits-Christoph et al., 1988). I discuss the tracking of a problem focus in Chapter 4.

4. *Competency in applying technical strategies and tactics flexibly and*

creatively. This competency addresses the style of the clinician's activities. The therapist must be able to operate *flexibly* within the framework of some model of therapeutic process and change. By this I mean that therapeutic strategy remains consistent with the model, even as specific interventions are determined both by their congruence with the technical strategy and by the immediate contextual demands (Beutler, 1997). The dynamic–interpersonal model of therapeutic process invites a technical strategy that promotes a particular sort of inquiry that has three broad aims: (a) progressively greater comprehension of the content, function, purposes, and history of salient maladaptive interpersonal patterns; (b) acquisition or enhancement of certain interpersonal problem-solving skills, and; (c) fostering of specific constructive interpersonal experiences. The disciplined implementation of a theory-driven technical strategy coupled with the flexible choice of specific interventions culminates in the quintessential therapeutic skill: the ability to *improvise* in response to unique therapeutic contexts. I discuss the flexible use of technical strategies and tactics to promote specific change processes in Chapters 5 and 6.

5. *Competency in relationship management.* The therapist must possess a set of skills that enables him or her effectively to manage vicissitudes in the interpersonal process that may occur during the course of a therapeutic relationship. The mutual involvement of patient and therapist assuredly constitutes a form of intimacy within the constraints of a professional arrangement. As with any intimate relationship, there are ups and down in the therapeutic dyad. The down periods can be quite tense. In addition, there is a significant potential challenge inherent in many therapeutic relationships. Anyone who genuinely requires psychotherapeutic intervention probably has significant difficulties in interpersonal relating, at least temporarily, regardless of symptoms. Furthermore, interpersonal difficulties usually involve hostility, which can often be very subtly expressed. The patient may convey hostility in a manner that pulls for a reciprocal reaction from the therapist—who is, after all, only human. The result is "negative process"; that is, patient–therapist interactions that are characterized by complimentary hostility, in which the provocative action of one party (i.e., the patient) has a high probability of evoking a reciprocal hostile reaction from the other party (i.e., the therapist) (Kiesler, 1996). Whether termed "negative transference and countertransference," or "vicious circles" (Wachtel, 1993) or "cyclical maladaptive interpersonal patterns" (Strupp & Binder, 1984), I and others propose that negative process is a primary impediment to therapeutic change in all forms of

psychotherapy and is a widely underestimated factor in therapeutic
relationships (Binder & Strupp, 1997a). Accordingly, therapists must
develop a set of skills associated with identifying and effectively resolving episodes of negative process, if they arise. The core of these
skills involves forms of self-monitoring within the flow of interpersonal process. The concept of negative process and the skills associated
with managing it are discussed in Chapter 7.

The discussions in the chapters to follow include a description of
each competency, clinical illustrations of it and the identification of
specific therapeutic skills and underlying generic skills associated with
each. In Chapter 8, Karishma Patel and I discuss the unique skills involved in terminating therapy. Chapter 9 addresses the topic of psychotherapy training and elucidates significant problems in training
that have been identified as a consequence of research using manual-
guided therapist training formats.

NOTES

1. This view is increasingly held by psychotherapy researchers (who depend
   on policymakers for research funds), teachers (who are pressured by ac-
   crediting organizations to promote only treatments or interventions that
   are empirically supported), and practitioners (who, for the most part, are
   feeling coerced into accepting this view in order to get reimbursed by third-
   party payers).
2. It should be kept in mind that the dose–effect data represent aggregate results reflecting the hypothetically average therapist. It is conceivable that
   the more skillfully you conduct therapy, the more efficient you can be.
   Whereas developing skill is a broad, ambitious goal, there is some empirical support for a specific, tangible way to improve therapeutic efficiency
   and effectiveness. Therapists who solicit feedback from their patients about
   the patients' responses to treatment sessions can potentially enhance outcomes and, at least, improve efficiency by reducing treatment failures or
   dropouts, particularly with difficult patients. Patient responses to treatment sessions—in the form of evaluations of symptoms, functioning, and
   the state of the therapeutic alliance—can be obtained from easy to administer self-report measures after each treatment session (Lambert, Whipple, et
   al., 2001; Lambert et al., 2002).

2

Competency 1

The Use of Theoretical Models of Personality, Psychopathology, and Therapeutic Process to Guide the Conduct of Psychotherapy

There is one requisite competence to which all other therapeutic competencies are anchored. This fundamental competence is comprised of congruent conceptual models of personality, psychopathology, and therapeutic process. First, therapists must have some theory about how individuals function within an interpersonal milieu; in other words, a theory of personality that is applicable to the psychotherapeutic setting. Second, therapists must have some theory about how functioning within an interpersonal milieu can go awry; that is, a theory of psychopathology that views human problems in a way that is relevant to psychotherapeutic actions. Third, therapists must have a theory about the cognitive, affective, and behavioral processes activated during patient–therapist interactions; in other words, a theory of therapeutic process. Finally, therapists' theories about therapeutic process must contain principles concerning how personality change is promoted.

Such a theoretical framework guides therapists' approach to clinical data, including what data to look for and how to understand them. A guiding theory enhances therapists' pattern recognition skills, so that they are more accurate and efficient at identifying, extracting, and organizing patterns of information into a psychotherapeutically useable case formulation of a central issue or theme. Similarly, they are more efficient at designing intervention strategies that utilize their conceptualization of the therapeutic process in a manner that effectively addresses patients' unique conditions. Problem-focused case formulations are more precise and minimize trial-and-error technical interventions, thereby promoting time-sensitive or time-effective treatment.

Each of the major theoretical orientations toward personality, psychopathology, and psychotherapy has an enormous corpus of theoretical writings. Therapists can attend to only a minute portion of this information when conducting therapy. In order to drive a car, you do not have to be aware of all of the knowledge that you may possess about automobiles. The vast majority of the time you use only the small portion of this information that is essential for actually driving at that point in time. The same process of selective activity applies to other complex performances. Whether in sports, music, other professions, trades, etc., skillful behavior is partly characterized by intuitively correct actions. In other words, the behavior of competent and expert practitioners within any given field is largely based on automatized patterns of action that require a minimum of deliberate thought. As discussed in Chapter 1, the knowledge and skills guiding the performer are largely tacit, a knowing-in-action (Schon, 1983; Sternberg & Horvath, 1999) or procedural knowledge (Glaser, 1989; Holyoak, 1991; Kihlstrom, 1987). This largely automatized knowledge guides behavior once the problem context has been comprehended. Given that procedural knowledge allows us to fly largely by autopilot, so to speak, how are the coordinates initially set and subsequently adjusted? In terms of our particular domain of interest, how is the changing therapeutic context understood?

Therapists must have a conscious cognitive map or "working model" of the immediate therapeutic situation, including just enough theory to comprehend the problem context and design intervention strategies, but not so much as to get in the way of attunement to the patient and spontaneous reactions to the changing context. Such a mental model is composed of a synopsis of theories that is sufficiently parsimonious to enable the therapist to manage it as a conceptual framework that is more or less consciously maintained. This mental model serves to sharpen rather than impede a clear view of the therapeutic setting and should guide the following therapist tasks:

1. Formulating a problem or issue to serve as the focus of treatment, including a hypothetical explanation of the origin of the problem and what sustains it over time.
2. Formulating treatment goals that are derived from the problem formulation.
3. Envisioning the nature of the therapeutic process (i.e.. facets of the patient–therapist interactions and relationship), including generic therapeutic change processes, obstacles to change, and the roles of therapist and patient.
4. Recognizing and managing salient features of the unique interpersonal process set in motion by this particular patient–therapist dyad.
5. Selecting a technical strategy that is appropriate for the particular patient with his or her particular problems.
6. Improvising in response to the unique circumstances of the particular therapeutic dyad but within the parameters set by the theoretical working model.

A PRACTICAL MODEL OF PERSONALITY FUNCTIONING

One way a therapist can represent a patient's personality in his or her mind's eye is in the form of self-representations and object-representations that are inextricably linked together by interaction scenarios characterized by affective tones (Hamilton, 1988; Mitchell, 1988). In other words, the building blocks of personality can be viewed as "interaction structures" that contain the self-representations associated with a sense of individual identity (Beebe, Lachman, & Jaffe, 1997; Sandler & Sandler, 1978). For example, say that a patient describes a situation in which she was at a social gathering but felt out of place and unwelcome. In response to the therapist's request for specifics about what made her feel this way, the patient describes how another person at the gathering spoke to her and made her feel tongue-tied, anxious, and unsure about what to say. Eventually, the other person became involved in a conversation with someone else, which the patient interpreted as a lack of interest in her. The therapist continues to query the patient to obtain further details about this interpersonal event, because details will help the therapist construct a more vivid mental picture of the patient's interaction with the other person. The picture constructed by the therapist portrays the other person as someone trying to make casual social conversation with the patient, who is not able to respond well. The therapist's impression is that the other person could have misinterpreted the patient's shyness as lack of interest in continuing the conversation. Through this inquiry process, the therapist constructs a mental model of an interpersonal scenario in which the patient, through her own behavior and assumptions about the intentions and attitudes of others, unwittingly contributed to her feeling that others were rejecting her.

Psychological "structures" are ingrained patterns of mental activity that are slow to form and slow to change. From the perspective of a therapist attempting to understand and work with a patient, it is easier to comprehend these psychological patterns in terms of narrative interpersonal themes. These interactional structures or self-object representational units occupy the foreground of personality, whereas cognitive and perceptual processes are conceived of as occupying the background of personality, where they function as information processors of the content contained in the interaction structures.

The interactional structures that characterize each personality are the product of the internalization of interpersonal experiences. From the moment of birth on, the transactions with others, particularly those upon whom the individual relies for protection and physical and emotional sustenance (i.e., "significant others"), are internalized and fundamentally influence the organization and content of the emerging personality structure. There always are reciprocal influences during transactions between two individuals. Even in earliest infancy, the temperament and constitutionally determined interactional style of the infant influence the caretaker's responses and set in motion particular transactional patterns, resulting in the internalization of particular interpersonal experiences.[1] Internalized childhood experiences form the foundation of personality structure, which, in turn, influences the nature of later internalizations. Later internalizations, however, can modify internal structures that were the product of earlier experiences (Mitchell, 1988).

The internalized representations of interpersonal experiences approximate what actually occurs *if* the individual is not under significant interpersonal stress at the time. For example, a child's experience of her mother gently admonishing her for some misbehavior would be encoded in the child's memory as a relatively accurate representation of the interaction: a lesson in disapproved behavior in the context of a loving relationship. On the other hand, stress, particularly extended interpersonal stress—what Pine (1990) calls "strain trauma"—is likely to impair cognitive and perceptual functions, resulting in misrepresentations, misinterpretations, or outright distortions of the interpersonal occurrences that are internalized. Chronic interpersonal stress with persons of emotional significance will lead to misperceived and distorted experiences that, when internalized, have significant influence on the development (or maldevelopment) of personality structure. For example, a child is chronically depressed and anxious because his mother is emotionally unavailable to nurture him from time to time. She suffers from recurrent depressive episodes, during which she is unable to adequately respond to her child's emotional needs. The child, in turn, repeatedly internalizes these episodes interpreting these experiences as abandonment of an unlovable child by a rejecting, neglectful mother. He grows up to be a wary, anxious adult, who views himself as unlovable and others as fickle in their offers of intimacy.

The interactional structures that comprise the foundation of personality are composites of multiple discrete internalized experiences that share common narrative elements. The common narrative element may be, for example, a particular person, such as a mother; or a particular person associated with a particular sentiment, such as a critical father; or a particular set of reciprocal roles, such as the self as subordinate to an authority figure. In other words, an interactional structure is one type of schema, one category of generalized knowledge or pattern of information. If you could take a series of photographs depicting various scenes of people interacting, in which all the scenes involve a common interpersonal theme (e.g., rejection, neglect, approval, hostility, etc.), and synthesize them into a composite photograph that represents a prototype of this theme, then you would have a visual analogy of an interpersonal schema. These personality structures or schemas are not directly accessible to conscious awareness (Horowitz, 1998; Orlinsky & Geller, 1993). They contribute, however, to derivative self-object representational units (Horowitz, 1998) that can be maintained in conscious awareness.

As noted previously, in any interpersonal encounter, an individual makes sense of, and is guided by a cognitive map or internal working model of the situation (Bowlby, 1988; Horowitz, 1998). According to Bowlby (1988):

> The function of these models is to simulate happenings in the real world, thereby enabling the individual to plan his behavior with all the advantages of insight and foresight. The more adequate and accurate the simulation . . . the better adapted the behavior based on it is

likely to be. . . . Because these models are in constant use, day in and day out, their influence on thought, feeling, and behavior becomes routine and largely outside of awareness. (pp. 165–166)

The core of this working model is a self-object representational unit, a "structured role relationship" (Horowitz, 1998), composed of a self-representation with particular personal and role characteristics, an object-representation with respective characteristics, and an anticipated sequence of interactions with a particular affective tone. This structured role relationship is the product of the combined influences of (1) the interpersonal themes representing schemas activated because they have some thematic relevance to the immediate interpersonal context, as well as (2) information from the immediate context. Structured role relationships that are part of a working model are potentially accessible to conscious awareness. "Outside of awareness" could be termed "nonconscious"; the term is intended to convey the limited amount of information that the mind can consciously manage at any given time. "Outside of awareness" also could refer to the "dynamic unconscious," where content is actively kept from awareness because of its disturbing nature (Bowlby, 1969). A working model also includes the cognitions, affects, and mental organizing processes that are associated with the core structured role relationship. An adaptive working model is flexible and can be modified by immediate feedback as the interaction unfolds, even though it is the product of combining schematic themes and direct observations of the current situation in which the person is engaged (Horowitz, 1998).

The salient themes that characterize a person's internal working models are reflected in the distinguishing features of his or her personality and interpersonal style. An individual's characteristic pattern of interacting with others tends to evoke a circumscribed, reciprocal range of reactions from others. These reactions, in turn, tend to reinforce the likelihood that the original interpersonal actions will be repeated, because they tend to fulfill the expectations of the instigator of the original actions. For example, one person does something caring and considerate for another person, expecting that this act will be appreciated. The recipient of the thoughtful act does indeed respond with an appreciative attitude and a reciprocal act of kindness. The first person's expectation was fulfilled, thus making it more likely that he or she will repeat the type of action that evoked the consequent appreciative reaction in a similar future situation. Through such complimentary transactions, an interpersonal style tends to become self-perpetuating (Benjamin, 1993; Kiesler, 1996; Strupp & Binder, 1984; Wachtel, 1993).

Personality structures and the corresponding interpersonal patterns that have been established in the past exert a powerful influence on how new interpersonal situations are perceived, interpreted, and responded to. New information is modified as it is assimilated into expectations about the world. On the other hand, exposure to new patterns of information, especially if repeated, should result in modification of existing schemas and corresponding interpersonal patterns, in order to accommodate the new information. A healthy personality is defined by a balance between these processes of assimilation and accommodation. In turn, such a balance contains both stability as well as the capacity for flexible responses to new experiences (Piaget, 1967).

Why do we construct internal working models to guide behavior in interpersonal situations? Because they enable us to connect with others. Bowlby (1969) took an evolutionary perspective in which he postulated the existence of biologically ingrained behavioral systems whose purpose is to achieve and maintain physical proximity to caretakers, in order to ensure protection from predators and other dangers. Predating Bowlby's attachment theory, British object relations theorists had posited an inherent motivational striving for interpersonal relatedness, experienced as a yearning for intimacy (Fairbairn, 1952). The American interpersonal psychiatrist Harry Stack Sullivan (1954) theorized that a sense of security, produced by harmonious interpersonal interactions, constitutes the fundamental human motivation. Along the same lines, British analysts Sandler and Sandler (1978) stated that motivation is defined as a "wished for interaction" that is imposed upon an interpersonal situation in order to achieve a sense of well-being. This state of well-being is the subjective indication that the relationship is securely harmonious and capable of providing emotional sustenance. Whereas relatedness is the primary focus in relational theories of motivation, Safran and Muran (2000) have pointed out another motivational theme in the literature: the striving for "agency," that is, for effectiveness, mastery, autonomy, and self-sufficiency. Safran and Muran describe the existential dialectic tension and potential for conflict that exist between the motives for relatedness and for independence. From infancy onward, taking independent action in the world is possible only if the individual is confident that a "secure base" of interpersonal intimacy awaits his or her return (Bowlby, 1988; Mahler, Pine, & Bergman, 1970).

The intrapsychic motives involving relatedness and agency are represented in the interpersonal arena by two corresponding dimensions of behavior. Interpersonal theorists have posited, and researchers have demonstrated, that all interpersonal behavior can be defined as some blend of two dimensions: the quality of affiliation, between love and hate; and the quality of interdependence, between control and submission. All interactions can be viewed as derivatives and variations of a fundamental negotiation about the affective tone and degree of intimacy that will define the relationship (Benjamin, 1993; Kiesler, 1996; Safran & Muran, 2000).

Thus, from a relational perspective personality is conceptualized as an interaction between internal psychological structures (i.e., schemas comprising interactional structures, as well as their derivative structured role relationships and working models) and patterned interpersonal interactions or relationship styles. Personality functioning is conceived of as the product of a system of reciprocally reinforcing internal structures, patterned interpersonal actions, and patterned evoked reactions from others. Wachtel has termed such a reciprocally reinforcing system "cyclical psychodynamics" (Wachtel, 1993).[2]

A PRACTICAL MODEL OF PSYCHOPATHOLOGY

Currently, the predominant language for discussing psychopathology is "descriptive psychopathology": the categorization of disturbed mental functioning by (more or less observable) signs and symptoms. The categorical system currently in use in the United States is codified in the fourth edition of the *Diagnostic and Statistical Manual of Mental Disorders* (American Psychiatric Association, 1994). Subsequent editions will undoubtedly be published, but the conceptual strategy will remain unchanged. In order to maximize diagnostic reliability, conceptions of psychopathology are limited to broad, relatively superficial descriptions of psychological impairments and distress. The strategy of descriptively categorizing "mental disorders" is often compared to taxonomies in fields such as biology and botany. The point is made that categorization is the first step in organizing the data in a field of inquiry, as a prerequisite to efforts at systematic explanation (Widiger, 1997). Nevertheless, there are serious limitations to a descriptive system for dealing with psychological disorders. The descriptions are as broad and far removed from individual persons as are the categorical systems in ethnology that characterize various cultures but reveal relatively little about any individual representing a particular culture.

The major theories of personality and psychopathology (e.g., psychodynamic, cognitive-behavioral, interpersonal) attempt to provide general explanations and treatment guidelines for disturbed functioning. These theories share several common themes concerning psychopathology:

1. The primary pantheoretical theme involves psychological rigidity of some sort. In the relational model presented here, there is a rigid, recurrent use of a limited variety of internal working models regarding interpersonal relations, with a corresponding constricted range of rigidly enacted interpersonal patterns. In this framework, mental health is characterized by use of a relatively wide variety of interpersonal working models that are flexibly adapted to changing interpersonal contexts. Furthermore, over time, changing life circumstances are accompanied by gradual modifications in the individual's repertoire of internal working models, reflecting changes in underlying interpersonal schemas. By contrast, ossified interpersonal schemas result in rigid working models, with the consequent intrusion of inappropriate interpersonal scripts into contemporaneous situations (Beck et al., 1979; Bowlby, 1988; Horowitz, 1998). For example, a man in his early 50s was getting repeated reprimands at work because of his frequent quarrels with his colleagues. His position required that he work with his colleagues as a troubleshooter on technical problems in his company's operation. However, he unwittingly superimposed on this interpersonal situation an old family pattern in which he felt ignored by his parents, whom he perceived as favoring his siblings. As a result, at work he felt unsupported by his superiors and experienced his colleagues as obstructing and demanding. He interpreted their offers of help with joint responsibilities as intrusions, to which he responded with irritation.

2. A second pantheoretical theme refers to a relatively restricted range of mental and/or behavioral actions. In the relational model presented here, a limited repertoire of rigidly enacted internal working models and corresponding interpersonal patterns contributes to a restricted range of responses from others. Others are inadvertently recruited into assuming roles in the maladaptive scenarios being unconsciously enacted by the individual. These reactions by others tend to reinforce the individual's interpersonal expectations, in turn reinforcing relevant interpersonal schemas. The result is a self-perpetuation of

vicious interpersonal cycles (Safran & Segal, 1990; Strupp & Binder, 1984; Wachtel, 1993). In the example cited above, the man's colleagues complained to their supervisor about his irritability and also complained directly to him. He, in turn, interpreted their reactions as unsupportive and demanding, thus reinforcing his initial anachronistic expectations.

3. A third pantheoretical theme refers to the distressing content of subjective experience. In the relational model presented here, the restricted range of internal working models and corresponding interpersonal patterns represent narrative themes that are inevitably distressing. Consequently, the interpersonal scenarios and relationships in which the person experiences him- or herself as a character or participant are colored by conflict, tension, uncertainty, and distress. Two broad categories of distressing experiences that have been associated with mental disorders are (1) fears and anxieties about possible internal and external threats to one's psychological and physical well-being (associated with anxiety disorders), and (2) depression, despair, and dejection over an anticipated lack of support from others, self-devaluation, and a sense of helplessness and hopelessness (associated with depressive disorders; Beck et al., 1979; Beck & Emery, 1985). Most affective, vegetative, and behavioral symptoms can be explained as responses to these distressing prototypic interpersonal scenarios. The man described above complained of chronic dysphoric mood associated with a sense that people did not like him and that his life was going nowhere.

4. The psychopathological working models and interpersonal patterns do not necessarily mean that rigid and anachronistic inter nalized patterns have been "frozen in time" and are literally reenacted (Mitchell, 1988). The past exerts an influence in more subtle, indirect ways. As mentioned above, schemas contribute to the establishment of temporary internal working models used to comprehend the immediate situation. These internal working models and their corresponding interpersonal patterns are pathological to the extent that they represent distressing interpersonal themes and inappropriate generalizations to contemporaneous situations that contain even a kernel of commonality with the characteristics of the activated, prototypic interpersonal schemas. It is assumed that a schema can be activated if its content overlaps with the interpersonal themes pervading the immediate interpersonal situation. The specific combination of schemas that is activated is impossible to predict. Psychopathological schemas, like pathological internal working models, are characterized

by disturbing interpersonal themes and maladaptive interpersonal coping strategies. They are easily activated, with very little content overlap with the immediate context, and, as mentioned above, are relatively impervious to change. In the example of the man with problems at work, there was little similarity between his childhood family situation and the circumstances at his job. What appeared to strike a resonant chord was that, in both situations, he did not feel that he received adequate guidance and support from authority figures: in his family the perceived negligence came from his parents, whereas at work it came from his supervisor.

5. A final theme refers to conflict, whether intrapsychic, interpersonal, or both (as in the relational model). Classic psychoanalytic theory conceptualizes intrapsychic conflict in terms of biologically based wishes and their derivatives that are opposed by internalized social prohibitions (Mitchell & Black, 1995). Object relations theory represents a transition between a purely intrapsychic conception of conflict and an interpersonal view. In object relations theory conflict is viewed in terms of internal structural "units" composed of self and object representations; different self-object units represent conflicting wishes (e.g., "I am a kind and trusting person" conflicts with "I am an assertive person who can succeed in this competitive world"), or a need or wish associated with a self-representation is linked to some rejecting, disapproving, or otherwise negative reaction of the object-representation (e.g., "If I am confident other people will view me as arrogant") (Mitchell & Black, 1995). Interpersonal theories view conflict in interpersonal terms: The actions of one person evoke negative reactions from another (Kiesler, 1996). Relational theories, which I draw upon to explain behavior, combine aspects of object relations and interpersonal theories to explain conflict: That is, they link dysfunctional mental activity with maladaptive interpersonal behavior. An individual has a dysfunctional mental working model of interpersonal relations when what appears to be, or is, a benign wish, intention, or anticipated act is expected to evoke a reaction in others that will cause the person distress or harm. In turn, the person's overt behavior is guided by the dysfunctional mental working model; he or she unwittingly (i.e., unconsciously) orchestrates a scenario in which the other person is recruited into playing a role that, in self-defeating fashion, fulfills his or her expectations of dissatisfying interpersonal relations. This unhappy interpersonal experience reinforces the psychopathological schemas that underlie his or her dysfunctional working model and corresponding maladaptive interpersonal behavior. An example of

this process is the woman, described above, who anticipated rejection in social situations. Her expectations contributed to her inability to carry on a conversation at a social gathering. The person to whom she was trying to talk mistook her shyness as a lack of interest in the conversation and, consequently, moved on. She interpreted this act as disinterest in her—which is what she expected and feared all along. It is likely that in the next social encounter, she will be even more anxious and inhibited.

A CLINICAL ILLUSTRATION OF THE THEORIES OF PERSONALITY AND PSYCHOPATHOLOGY

Ms. Brody was a successful professional woman, unmarried, who had a network of good friends but also strongly desired a satisfying intimate relationship with a man. For a long time Ms. Brody believed that the source of her unhappiness in romance stemmed from her lack of self-confidence, which, in turn, stemmed from her assumption that she was physically unattractive and had an unappealing personality. She held this conviction in spite of having a pleasant appearance combined with exceptional intelligence and sense of humor. Ms. Brody had grown up in a stable family, with parents who showed their love through their reliability but who were unable overtly to express loving feelings. At times her mother could be nurturing and supportive but had always put subtle pressure on her daughter to somehow make up for the nurturing that she had lacked from her own neglectful mother. Ms. Brody's mother had been demonstrably upset when her daughter had moved to another part of the country. Her father reinforced a sense of obligation for her to nurture her mother (e.g., "Why don't you come and visit, because your mother would love to go shopping with you?"). She also felt an obligation to take care of her father. Although he had a successful career, he had poor relationships with his family, few friends, and was excruciatingly uncomfortable with feelings and personal topics. Outside of his family, this discomfort was effectively masked by an interpersonal style that combined a certain stiff formality with a focus on the interests of the other person. Ms. Brody's mother would reinforce her daughter's sense of obligation to avoid causing her father discomfort by repeatedly warning her daughter not to disturb her father with anything upsetting. Not surprisingly, Ms. Brody developed a prepotent interpersonal schema of a significant other, particularly men, that was a composite of features from both her mother and father: Men are interpersonally needy and emotionally very fragile. She had contradictory self-schemas associated with the schema of men: on the one hand, an unappealing, unlovable self-schema associated with an expectation of disappointing the other; on the other hand, a smart, successful self-schema associated with an expectation of being stifled or engulfed by obligations toward others.

These interpersonal schemas influenced the internal working models she used to comprehend her interactions with men and to guide her transactions with them. One interpersonal pattern involved her worry that "time was passing," and she still had not experienced a pleasurable romantic relationship. She saw herself as unappealing and tended to make connections with men who were already involved or who were incompatible with her values and interests. When things did not work out and she felt spurned, her self-image as unlovable was reinforced, as was her image of men as inevitably "put off" by her. On the other hand, when a man who appeared compatible expressed an interest in her, Ms. Brody became critical of even minor foibles she detected in him. She was exquisitely sensitive to any indication of emotional neediness in the man, and tended to misinterpret expressions of his desire for intimacy as early warnings of stifling restrictions, which she anticipated he would place on her autonomy. She would react with emotional withdrawal. The man, in turn, would eventually back off, and the relationship would ultimately dissolve, leaving Ms. Brody again feeling lonely and unloved.

The maladaptive interpersonal pattern is the observable portion of interlocked and reciprocally reinforcing intrapersonal and interpersonal elements: Ms. Brody's rigid and contradictory self-schemas and schemas of men; the resulting rigid and constricted internal working models of herself in relationships with men; her corresponding rigid and restricted repertoire of interpersonal behavior with potential male suitors; and the restricted range of evoked reactions from those suitors. All of these elements combined to produce a self-perpetuating cycle of distressing and impaired interpersonal functioning in her personal relationships with men.

A USEABLE THEORY OF THERAPEUTIC PROCESS

In *Psychotherapy in a New Key: A Guide to Time-Limited Dynamic Psychotherapy* (Strupp & Binder, 1984), we presented a point of view that is further elaborated in this book. Specific technical recommendations are impossible to make in advance, because the impact of any technical intervention will be influenced by its immediate interpersonal meaning to the patient, which in turn is determined by the immediate interpersonal context. As a guide to therapist action, Strupp and I recommended a conceptual model of the *therapeutic process*, a term that refers to the interpersonal dynamics (i.e., influences) emerging out of the ongoing interactions between patient and therapist. These interactions are influenced by and reciprocally influence the internal working models guiding the patient and therapist. A theory of therapeutic process should specify the interpersonal facets postulated to be part of the process, the roles of each participant, the postulated agents of therapeutic change, and any anticipated potential obstacles to change. For a theory of therapeutic process to be useful, it must be a succinct conceptual framework that can be (1) stored in the background of the therapist's awareness and (2) regularly accessed to guide performance during the course of a therapy session. If a therapist is using the relational theories of personality and psychopathology presented above, then a theory of therapeutic process must elucidate how change occurs in a relational model of personality.

The interpersonal medium for therapeutic process is the "real relationship." This term refers to the realistic reasons why a patient and a therapist get together. The patient seeks help with psychological problems from a professional who is viewed as an expert in these matters and who is assumed to be trustworthy (an assumption based on anything from a referral by someone who is known and trusted, to reputation, to blind faith). The psychotherapist views him- or herself as a professional who offers a service to patients within the parameters of agreed-upon arrangements, even if this commitment entails a certain amount of emotional stress and strain (Greenson & Wexler, 1969; Strupp & Binder, 1984). In a time-limited psychotherapy guided by relational principles, the patient is expected to come to each session prepared to talk candidly about any topic that, in the patient's view, is relevant to the agreed-upon problem focus. If the patient does not have such a topic in mind, then he or she is encouraged to talk about anything that comes to mind. This strategy is based on the fundamental psychoanalytic principle of "psychic determinism," which states that the patient's spontaneous verbalizations will reveal prepotent, affectively charged themes. The therapist's role is to offer his or her attention and expertise for the purpose of facilitating a therapeutically productive dialogue. This goal is accomplished through a variety of interventions, including observations, questions, and interpretations. In addition, the therapist attempts to minimize the influence of his or her own needs and desires, unless they can contribute positively to the therapeutic relationship (e.g., the desire to be an effective therapist).

In order for a patient and therapist to work together effectively, a therapeutic alliance must be established and maintained. How this facet of therapeutic process operates in time-limited psychotherapies has been conceptualized in a variety of ways (Safran & Muran, 1998) and is discussed in greater detail in Chapter 6. A therapeutic alliance involves an explicit agreement between therapist and patient to *collaborate* on working toward resolution of the patient's problems. This collaboration is based on an agreement, sometimes achieved through negotiation, about the goals of therapy and the tasks required of each party to reach these goals. At least equally important, the alliance is based on an emotional bond of liking and trust that quickly grows out of the experiences of a patient and therapist with each other. The therapeutic alliance derives primarily from the real relationship between patient and therapist, although it may be augmented by positive transference and countertransference (what Freud, 1912/1955, referred to as "unobjectionable positive transference").

Ideally, the alliance would remain consistently strong. However, it has been demonstrated that "alliance ruptures" can occur during the course of treatment (Safran & Muran, 2000). From a relational perspective, these strains and breaches in the therapeutic alliance are the manifestation of prepotent maladaptive interpersonal patterns of interaction (i.e., transference and countertransference responses; Safran & Muran, 2000; Strupp & Binder, 1984). An early and still widely held view of the therapeutic alliance is that, if established, its positive influence remains largely static over the course of treatment (Horvath & Greenberg, 1994). A recently proposed opposite view, stemming from empirical studies of therapeutic process, is that the alliance changes literally from interaction to interaction (Henry & Strupp, 1994). An alternative to either of these extreme views, and more consistent with the concept of alliance ruptures and repairs, is a conception of the therapeutic alliance as comparable to a malleable solid. From this view the alliance is usually stable, but it is also vulnerable to changing in response to the vicissitudes of interpersonal interactions. The speed and direction of change (from firm to strained or ruptured alliance, or vice versa) is determined by the strength and quality of the preceding and immediate interactions (Binder & Strupp, 1997b; Safran & Muran, 2000).

Although not always stated explicitly, how a clinician views the alliance's susceptibility to vicissitudes is associated with his or her con-ception of the role of the alliance in therapeutic change. In discussions of brief psychotherapy, there are big differences of opinion about this role. For example, brief psychodynamic therapists who apply a self psychology framework assume that positive psychological change results from "transmuting internalizations" of interactions during which the therapist demonstrates empathy with the patient's distress (Ser-uya, 1997). The implicit assumption is that, at least in the relatively short time span of a brief treatment, a competent therapist can be con-sistently warm, interested, and empathic, thereby contributing to a consistently strong alliance. There is compelling evidence, however, scattered throughout the clinical and empirical literature, that it is not as easy for a therapist to maintain this sort of stance as is frequently assumed (Binder & Strupp, 1997a).

In their brief relational therapy, Safran and Muran (2000) recog-nize the difficulties that therapists can encounter in attempting to maintain a warm and empathic stance. This recognition leads them to focus on what they consider to be the inevitable ruptures in any thera-peutic alliance. They posit that in brief treatment positive change is most effectively conduced by focusing on whatever alliance strains and ruptures occur in the patient–therapist relationship. The process of resolving these alliance ruptures, they contend, will positively influ-ence the patient in whatever areas of his or her life are problematic. Here, the explicit assumptions are that (1) alliance ruptures inevitably occur and (2) are necessary requisites to positive therapeutic change.

In my clinical experience, I have found that alliance ruptures may or may not occur in brief psychotherapy, perhaps because of its brevity. If they do occur, they must be resolved; if they do not occur, therapeu-tic work can proceed just fine, because there are effective methods of producing positive psychological change that do not rely on the reso-lution of alliance ruptures. Time-limited therapists have emphasized the importance of rapidly establishing and consistently maintaining a therapeutic alliance for the obvious reason that time is at a premium. It has been assumed, therefore, that alliance ruptures in these forms of treatment will be more disruptive than in open-ended treatments, be-cause there is less time available to deal with them (Safran & Muran, 1998). On the other hand, what has been overlooked in briefer thera-pies is that although an alliance has formed, significant ruptures may not have time to develop. An alliance rupture is a form of tension or conflict that occurs in the course of the development of a relationship. When both participants have reasonably good capacities for interpersonal relating, then a new interaction or relationship is likely to have an initial "honeymoon" phase during which expectations are largely positive (Piper et al., 1993). Sometimes relationships involve brief but intense liaisons, which can have a profound and enduring impact, but during which a potential for interpersonal conflict may not have time to ignite. Thus various forms of relatively brief relationships may run their course with little, if any, conflict. Similarly, relatively brief therapies (i.e., less than 25 sessions) may not evidence significant alliance ruptures. In other words, relatively brief therapeutic relationships may last long enough to effectively examine a patient's interpersonal problems in outside relationships but may not last long enough for those problems to significantly impact the therapeutic relationship (Connolly et al., 1996).[3]

On the other hand, there are individuals who enter any relationship, including a therapeutic encounter, with a deep-seated and pervasive mistrust in, or pessimism about, what other people have to offer. Accordingly, they tend to be resistant to entering into a therapeutic alliance (Piper et al., 1993). It may take a relatively lengthy period for even an embryonic alliance to form. Under these circumstances, the time constraints associated with briefer forms of therapy may be a serious, if not terminal, disadvantage. Between these two levels of potential for successful interpersonal relating is the majority of persons who enter a therapeutic relationship with high hopes but who may eventually experience distress toward, and a breakdown in effective collaboration with, their therapists.

Within the therapeutic relationship, the enactment of maladaptive patterns typically originates with the patient but may quickly ensnare the therapist. The result may be a strain or rupture in the therapeutic alliance. Discussions of alliance ruptures have an all-or-nothing tone; that is, if a maladaptive interpersonal pattern (i.e. transference–countertransference) is enacted, an alliance rupture ensues. Whereas in open-ended treatment a maladaptive interpersonal pattern enactment that goes undetected may inevitably gain in strength to the point of becoming an alliance rupture, the time constraints associated with briefer therapies may short-circuit this process. In other words, the influence of a maladaptive interpersonal pattern enactment on a therapeutic alliance may vary over time. One person may enter treatment and quickly enact a transference pattern that initiates an alliance strain or rupture. Another patient's maladaptive interpersonal pattern may not initiate an alliance rupture until later in treatment, or may not emerge at all during the course of a time-limited treatment. This view of the relationship between maladaptive interpersonal pattern enactments and therapeutic alliance has implications for the therapist's technical strategy, which are discussed in Chapters 5 and 6. A graphic representation of this model of therapeutic process is presented in Figure 2.1.

A CLINICAL ILLUSTRATION OF A TIME-LIMITED THERAPY WITHOUT A SIGNIFICANT ALLIANCE RUPTURE

Mrs. Price is in her mid-50s and happily married for the second time. She has no children from either marriage and has apparently reconciled herself to never having children. For approximately a year she has suffered from symptoms of anxiety and depression, including tension, emotional lability, sleep and concentration disturbances, fatigue, and diminished sexual interest. She has an extended family who are emotionally close. Several months before seeking therapy, Mrs. Price's mother suffered a stroke that caused serious cognitive and physical impairments. Consequently, her close relationship with her mother (e.g., "She was my best friend") was significantly altered. The precipitant for seeking therapy was increasing stress at her job. She had been an employee at a small company from its inception, and in her administrative position she had helped it grow to its current significantly

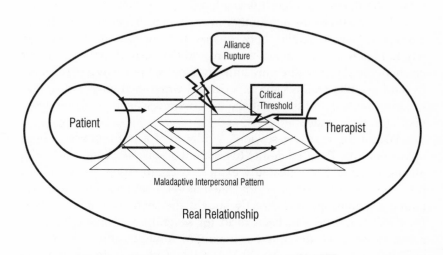

FIGURE 2.1. Model of therapeutic process.

larger size. When the company was small, the supervisors and employees related to each other like a family. Mrs. Price had an instrumental coordinating role, similar to the role she played in her own family of origin. As the company grew, new employees were added and relationships became more impersonal. For the last couple of years, Mrs. Price has had a supervisor with very high standards who relates to his employees in a stern and critical manner. Although she is very competent and usually avoided being targeted for his public criticisms, she no longer enjoyed her work. Recently he criticized her in front of her coworkers. Mrs. Price reacted by abruptly leaving work and taking a medical leave of absence due to the increase in her symptoms of anxiety and depression. She sought psychotherapy to resolve her symptoms and to obtain help in deciding whether or not to return to work. On the one hand, she felt an obligation to her company and coworkers to continue working (even though financially, she did not need to work); on the other hand, she no longer obtained any pleasure from her work. Mrs. Price was paralyzed with indecision.

Early in therapy a content focus was identified: the parallel between her ambivalence about her job and her ambivalent feelings about the current relationship with her mother. She felt an obligation to stay at her job even though she no longer enjoyed it. She felt a loyalty to her company and coworkers based on their history together, which had been very pleasurable and satisfying to her. Similarly, she felt an obligation to visit her mother in the nursing home where she now resided, even though it was a long, burdensome drive and emotionally stressful to see her mother in such an incapacitated condition. There also was a parallel between her wishful fantasy that her job would regain its original satisfaction, and the wishful fantasy that her mother would recuperate miraculously. Finally, there was a parallel between the guilty feelings she experienced when she thought of resigning from her job and the guilt she experienced whenever she ended a visit with her mother.

Within the first few sessions, evidence of a transference pattern appeared: Mrs. Price related to her male therapist in a coquettish, idealizing manner. She repeatedly expressed appreciation for her therapist's observations, reported that she felt very comforted in the therapeutic relationship, and directly sought the therapist's advice. Mrs. Price's father, who had been dead for several years and whom she sorely missed, was described as having high morals and integrity, but was also very authoritative, to the point of being domineering. Attempts to examine Mrs. Price's experience of the relationship with her therapist produced nothing but appreciative sentiments, and several attempts to draw parallels between her wish to rely heavily on her therapist's opinions and her lost relationship with her father fell on deaf ears. Mrs. Price appeared much more invested in experiencing the security of relating to her therapist in a trusting, supportive, and somewhat eroticized manner than in examining the nature of the relationship. She did, however, resonate to the parallel that her therapist drew between her past desire to please her father by succeeding in school and work and her desire to please her supervisor at work and avoid his displeasure by resigning.

During the course of therapy, which lasted 16 sessions, her mother's physical condition deteriorated and the content focus of treatment shifted to issues of death and loss, as Mrs. Price's anticipatory grieving increased. She evidenced an increased desire to receive guidance and support from her therapist, as well as to please him with "good behavior." During this time, she reported that she had decided to quit her job. Her mother's death accelerated her process of emotionally detaching from her job, as she assumed her characteristic role of coordinator of family activities around the funeral and its aftermath. She resonated to the therapist's observation that she reacted to grieving and turning her attention to new directions in her life with guilt, feeling as of she were letting everyone down: her supervisor and coworkers after announcing her resignation, and her family by not taking care of everyone's emotional needs. She did not, however, recognize these feelings in the relationship with her therapist, toward whom she continued to feel nothing but appreciation. The treatment terminated by mutual agreement after 16 sessions, with all symptoms resolved and the patient happily reporting that she and her husband had exciting plans for their immediate future.

Mrs. Price's strong positive alliance with her therapist was the foundation of the therapy. It was a major contributor to her receptiveness to his interventions, and it fueled her hope that together they could accomplish much. The somewhat idealized and eroticized tones associated with their positive alliance indicated the presence of transferential elements. The alliance may have been a bulwark against other issues, as well as a foundation of the immediate work, and there was no indication that any unresolved transference elements interfered with accomplishing the circumscribed (but for Mrs. Price, very important) goals of this brief therapy. Indeed, for the focused therapeutic aims of this treatment, the transferential elements present in the alliance may have may have contributed to the therapist's effectiveness.

GENERIC CHANGE PROCESSES

Interactions within a therapeutic relationship activate a therapeutic process. This process, in turn, is the medium within which positive changes occur in the patient. Although empirical research about the nature of the therapeutic process continues (e.g., Norcross, 2002; Orlinsky, Grawe, & Parks, 1994), the precise agents or processes of therapeutic change remain largely speculative. Each major theory of psychotherapy postulates certain change processes that are congruent with that theory. I refer to the change processes elucidated below as *generic* because they are postulated as operative in all major forms of psychotherapy and are derived from the major theories of therapy as well as from relevant principles in the cognitive sciences concerning knowledge and skill acquisition.

Cognitive Insight

Together, therapist and patient identify the latter's prepotent dysfunctional internal working models of interpersonal relationships, along with their corresponding maladaptive interpersonal patterns, which originate in the patient but potentially ensnare others, including the therapist. Patient and therapist then construct as precise a picture as possible of narrative themes that define these working models and interpersonal patterns, and they use this picture to help explain the meanings and functions of currently distressing and/or impairing mood, physical, and behavioral symptoms. Material to construct a picture of these internal working models and interpersonal patterns can be gathered through examination of the patient's recollections of current and past experiences outside of therapy. The most valid material, however, may sometimes be gathered from experiences within the patient–therapist relationship. The potential advantage of material from the therapeutic interaction is the modifying impact of immediate experience or current mental processes and behavior. To paraphrase the apocryphal aphorism: An *in vivo* experience is worth a thousand recollections or words.

The interpersonal themes that are developed as narrative substance for internal working models and interpersonal patterns are not assumed to reflect objective truths that have been discovered. Similarly, there are no historical "facts" to explain current patterns of psychological dysfunction, which can be dug up like Freud's famous metaphorical archeological relics. Such a positivistic epistemological position characterizes more orthodox psychodynamic, cognitive, and interpersonal theories. A "constructivist" epistemological position is more characteristic of a relational model of personality and therapy (Safran & Muran, 2000). A useable interpersonal theme is not "discovered" but, rather, jointly constructed by therapist and patient through their dialogues about the patient's current and past life, and sometimes from their firsthand experiences in the therapeutic relationship. The validity, or "narrative truth" (Spence, 1982), of an interpersonal theme is determined by how meaningful and plausible it is to both parties, and especially by how effective it is in facilitating the patient's conceptual reframing of his or her problems in a way that incites constructive action (Hoffman, 1983).

In psychodynamic, interpersonal, and cognitive theories, a positivistic epistemology of clinical data is associated with the more conservative technical strategy of delivering "correct" interventions at the right time (Kavanagh, 1995). From this perspective, the correctness of the content of an intervention is determined by how accurately the therapist has applied the cannons of his or her guiding theory to the clinical material of a particular case. The correct timing of the intervention also is usually defined by theory, but the guidelines are abstract and broad and tend to crumble into vagueness when actually used (at least in the case of psychodynamic theories). Often the therapist is left to rely on intuition or whim to determine the optimum moment to intervene. For example, a common principle for timing an interpretation in psychoanalytic therapy is to deliver it when the material is at the border of consciousness. But there is no precise method for determining when mental content is on this "border." In contrast, a constructivist epistemology of clinical data is associated with a technical strategy of encouraging a thematically productive dialogue. As discussed above, the correctness of the content of an intervention is determined by whether it effectively stimulates further dialogue and incites the patient to creative thought, affect, and action. Usually, there is no absolutely correct timing for any given intervention. The therapist can monitor the ongoing effectiveness of his or her interventions by evaluating the productiveness of the unfolding dialogue.[4]

Cognitive understanding involves the acquisition of declarative knowledge, which includes both autobiographical and abstract forms of knowledge. Autobiographical knowledge is a record of lived events; abstract knowledge consists of general concepts, principles, and rules about the world. As noted previously, declarative knowledge can be readily accessed in consciousness and comprises the major portion of a person's working model of which he or she is aware (Binder, 1999). When a patient calls his or her therapist to cancel a session, the relevant declarative knowledge includes generally agreed-upon courtesy as well as specifically agreed-upon rules for the therapeutic relationship. Declarative knowledge also is represented by the patient coming to understand, for example, that he is reluctant to disagree with his female therapist because he has uncritically assumed that she would be as intolerant of disagreement as his mother had been. This form of knowledge, by itself, is usually insufficient to produce changes in behavior. This limitation is reflected in the an Woody Allen scene in which he complains about being in psychoanalysis for 20 years without much change, so he resolves to give his analyst 10 more years to produce results before giving up on it.

Regardless of how intellectually meaningful it may be, declarative knowledge must be transformed into procedural knowledge. to serve as an effective change agent. Procedural knowledge guides when and how to apply declarative knowledge in real world situations. It develops from the repeated experience of applying concepts, principles, and prescriptions for action in daily life, and it consists of pairing propositions and concrete experiences with action strategies and rules, as well as appraisals of the consequences. To reiterate: Although procedural knowledge tends to operate automatically and outside of the person's conscious deliberation, it tacitly contributes to his or her working model of an interpersonal context (Binder, 1999). For example, the patient mentioned above knows (declarative knowledge) that if he cannot attend a therapy appointment, he should call to inform his therapist. He waits, however, until a few minutes before his appointment time to make this call (procedural knowledge). He consciously knows that his therapist has not given any indication that she is as critical as his mother, but this information does not get used in the current situation. Instead, his behavior continues to be directed by anachronistic procedural knowledge in the form of an internal model used as a child with his mother: He procrastinated about approaching mother with something that might irritate her in order to put off an unpleasant interchange. By calling at the last minute, however, the patient is likely to irritate his therapist, and her reaction, in turn, is likely to reinforce his preconception. In this fashion a maladaptive relational pattern is perpetuated. The concepts of declarative and procedural knowledge were developed by cognitive scientists to help explain the development of skill in various performance domains. They are relevant for discussing the process of change in psychotherapy when the essential goal is to perform more skillfully in interpersonal relationships.

Practice

The transformation of declarative knowledge into procedural knowledge requires practice in detecting the influence of dysfunctional internal working models and corresponding maladaptive interpersonal patterns. This practice can occur in any interpersonal situation between therapy sessions. The advantage of engaging in this sort of practice within the therapeutic relationship is the opportunity for immediate coaching by the therapist. The technical strategies of here-and-now transference–countertransference analysis (e.g., Strupp & Binder, 1984) or systematic metacommunicating about the therapeutic encounter (Safran & Muran, 2000) represent this form of immediate error-correcting feedback. This is a particularly powerful form of learning experience and is analogous to practicing a golf swing, or a musical instrument, or a medical procedure in the presence of a coach or teacher.

Practice in applying declarative knowledge acquired in therapy to appropriate outside interpersonal situations must be guided by the patient's own immediate appraisal of the situation and his or her performance. This real-world form of practice probably is most effective once the patient has acquired a sufficient level of skill in monitoring his or her interpersonal behavior and is clear about which maladaptive patterns of thinking and acting to note or censor. This self-monitoring skill is enhanced by practice within sessions, with feedback from the therapist, and between sessions in any and all forms of interaction, with delayed feedback from the therapist.

It appears, however, that in time-limited therapies many patients find it more meaningful to work on currently significant relationships outside of therapy than to use the therapy relationship (i.e., transference analysis) for this purpose (Connolly et al., 1999). One reason for this preference may be that the relatively short duration of the therapy relationship in time-limited therapies reduces the opportunity for the relationship to become as emotionally significant as other relationships in the patient's life, or to develop significant strains. There is no evidence that *in vivo* coaching by a therapist is more effective than retrospective examination, in the context of a strong therapeutic alliance, of relevant maladaptive interpersonal patterns enacted in outside relationships (Crits-Christoph et al., 1988; Piper et al., 1993; Silberschatz et al., 1986). In other words, although in many cases the development of interpersonal procedural knowledge may be optimized through practice in the therapeutic relationship, in many other cases substantial procedural knowledge may be acquired by relevant outside interpersonal encounters.

Creating New Behavior

First the patient and the therapist identify dysfunctional internal working models and corresponding maladaptive interpersonal patterns. Then they begin to practice detecting these models and patterns in relationships throughout the patient's life. This particular pattern recognition skill is but a prelude to developing healthier modes of thinking and relating. The old dysfunctional relational patterns must be deactivated, and new ways of thinking and acting must be rehearsed. The mental activity of initiating new ways of interpersonal relating represents the beginning of therapeutic change, and new reactions from significant others help consolidate new interpersonal patterns. New internal working models of interpersonal encounters and corresponding interpersonal patterns are developed that are more suited to current interpersonal realities and more responsive to changing conditions. These changes in the patient elicit more varied and satisfying reactions from others. Through this process new, benign interpersonal cycles are established and consolidated. The final result should be modification of relevant interpersonal schemas, thus producing a stable psychological foundation for therapeutic changes.

Internalization

Identifying dysfunctional working models and interpersonal patterns relies on two fundamental cognitive skills: interpersonal pattern recognition and self-reflection (Binder, 1999). The development of alternative, healthier cognitive and interpersonal patterns involves a creative cognitive process of internalization. As the new patterns of thinking and interacting are tried out and more satisfying interpersonal encounters ensue, these "corrective interpersonal experiences" are consolidated in the personality through the process of internalization (Greenberg & Mitchell, 1983). An episode of constructive, potentially mutative internalization takes place outside of therapy when the patient detects the operation of a maladaptive pattern in an interpersonal encounter, short-circuits the pattern, tries out a healthier mode of relating, and the other person responds in a more satisfying way than expected. Likewise, the internalization of a corrective interpersonal experience in the therapeutic relationship can occur in two ways:

1. Regardless of the area of the patient's life being examined, the experience of working collaboratively with the therapist in the context of a strong alliance is likely to be internalized. The positive experience with the therapist is usually sufficiently discrepant from what the patient expects in relationships with emotionally significant others that it is therapeutically mutative in its own right.
2. The process whereby patient and therapist successfully detect and resolve a therapeutic alliance rupture is likely to be internalized as a corrective interpersonal experience. Here again, this experience of collaborative conflict resolution with an emotionally significant other is usually discrepant from what the patient expects and, therefore, is therapeutically mutative (Safran & Muran, 2000).

Relational theories postulate that the process of internalizing of corrective interpersonal experiences, particularly within the therapeutic relationship, may be the primary factor in producing therapeutic change (Greenberg & Mitchell, 1983; Safran & Muran, 2000; Strupp & Binder, 1984). Internalization is an exceedingly subtle process that can not observed while it is occurring. Rather, it is inferred retrospectively by its assumed products (Orlinsky & Geller, 1993). For example, a patient reports greater satisfaction in a new interpersonal encounter as a result of being guided by a recent relevant discussion with his therapist, which occurred to him during the new encounter.

There is no information about how long it takes for a therapeutically effective internalization to occur. There are no average spans of time, no medians, no standard deviations in session or calendar units. It is assumed, however, that change resulting from internalization occurs gradually. Consequently, it is worth considering that the duration of time-limited therapies may sometimes not be sufficient to allow the internalization of corrective interpersonal experiences to have the major impact that is posited in open-ended treatments. It is possible that the achievement of cognitive understanding of dysfunctional patterns and practice in detecting and altering these patterns may set in motion a learning process that leads to the internalization of corrective interpersonal experiences, but these internalizations may not accumulate to a level that is therapeutically mutative until after the time-limited treatment has concluded. Therefore, it may be particularly important to develop the patient's self-reflection and pattern recognition skills to a level whereby he or she can continue to use them effectively after the therapist is no longer available as a coach. In order for the patient to acquire these skills in a relatively brief period of time, the therapist must actively promote their development by such efforts as directly and overtly discussing the importance of acquiring these skills for more successful living.

GENERIC SKILLS

The generic skills clients need to learn in the course of therapy are postulated by cognitive scientists to lay the foundation for effective actions across performance domains (Chi et al., 1988; Schon, 1983). As discussed above, the supraordinate goal of some forms of psychotherapy is to help the patient become more competent at managing interpersonal relationships. It follows, then, that the patient must develop those skills that comprise the foundation of any competent performance. Six generic skills appear to be necessary to facilitate the therapeutic change processes just enumerated:

Interpersonal Pattern Recognition

Interpersonal pattern recognition refers to the ability to recognize and extract evidence, from verbal and nonverbal communications, of interpersonal themes that influence the experiences and behaviors of oneself and others with whom one interacts. Specifically, the patient must learn to recognize prepotent interpersonal patterns that are associated with his or her internal working models and behavior with others.

Self-Reflection

Self-reflection refers to the ability to attend to one's own mental processes and actions, as well as to deliberate upon the information obtained from the act of self-observation.

Self-Monitoring

Self-monitoring refers to the ability to self-reflect over time. This mental activity is considered a separate skill because the achievement of consistent self-reflection over time, particularly during emotionally arousing interactions, takes more attention and concentration than a single act of self-reflection.

Reflection-on-Action

Reflection-on-action refers to the ability to pause during or after a particular interaction to evaluate it, with the aim of making necessary modifications or corrections. The purpose is to improve the effectiveness or satisfaction associated with an interaction (Schon, 1983). This is a higher-order skill that is based on the development of the first three skills.

Reflection-in-Action

Reflection-in-action is a refinement of reflection-on-action and reflects great proficiency in any performance domain, including interpersonal relationships. This is the ability to assess an ongoing interpersonal interaction and make necessary modifications or corrections during the course of the interaction, without interrupting it (Schon, 1983).

Improvisation

All of the preceding skills are required in order to achieve this highest-order capability, which is the hallmark of expertise in any performance domain, from the professions, to sports, to the arts. In the context of interpersonal relationships, improvisation refers to the ability of one party in a relationship to initiate a heretofore unthought of activity in order to overcome an impasse in the relationship caused by new circumstances. It is the ability to reframe problems and understandings and to adjust one's actions in response to changing contextual circumstances. The thematic richness and fluid nature of interpersonal interactions and relations create circumstances that are ambiguous, usually unpredictable in the particulars, and emotionally arousing. In other words, interpersonal interactions represent the ultimate in indeterminacy and therefore require the ability to improvise continuously to successfully manage them.[5]

Congruent with this model of therapeutic change processes is a role for the therapist that includes mentoring and coaching patients in the skills of managing interpersonal relations well. This type of role is considered too active and directive for the traditional psychodynamic therapist, who seeks to influence patients by providing empathic attunement to their subjective experiences—an attunement with which patients hopefully will identify (Messer & Warren, 1995). In contrast, I propose that the therapist must directly coach patients in the acquisition or improvement of the generic skills required to initiate generic therapeutic change processes as well as to achieve specific therapeutic goals. These generic skills are essentially the same skills that the psychotherapist must develop in order to effectively use therapeutic techniques, because the therapist, too, must be effective at managing the interpersonal relationship with his or her patients. Therefore, the competent therapist also teaches these generic skills by example. Perhaps a case vignette will illustrate this point.

Emily was a woman in her late 30s who had recently endured a painful divorce. Losses were particularly hard for her, because her parents had divorced when she was a small child, and she was raised by her withdrawn and depressed mother. Furthermore, when she was in her late teens, her father was killed in an automobile accident. Emily experienced real or symbolic losses (e.g., conflict with a loved one) as terrifying abandonment, which left her feeling alone in the world. She tended to relate to her older male therapist as a somewhat idealized authority figure, often trying to elicit his opinions about matters in her life. Although Emily's therapist was usually successful at minimizing her attempted recruitment into the role of a paternal advice giver (substituting for her dead father), he realized that frequently he did allow the sessions to run overtime by quite a bit. He shared this observation with Emily, and in the process of discussing why he allowed this to occur, they both agreed that Emily often felt that she did not have enough time during a session to talk about all that was on her mind. Her therapist suggested that perhaps he allowed the sessions to run overtime in order to protect Emily from feeling abandoned. He further suggested to her that perhaps he did not want her to see him like a father who had abandoned her. With this examination of what was transpiring between them, Emily appreciated, more than ever before, how much she had felt abandoned by her father when he divorced her mother and then when he died. This examination also provided Emily's therapist with an opportunity to model the generic skills of self-reflection and self-monitoring, and it provided Emily with a chance to practice them.

GENERIC OBSTACLES TO THERAPEUTIC CHANGE

There are several commonly encountered obstacles to therapeutic change, regardless of the unique characteristics specific to any particular therapeutic dyad.

Patient–Therapist Disagreement

There can be a disagreement between patient and therapist about what constitutes meaningful therapeutic goals and/or reasonable tasks for achieving the goals. These differences can be philosophical, cultural, or simply personal in nature. For example, a patient wants medication or specific behavioral interventions to remove a symptom, whereas the therapist is convinced that verbal exploration of the underlying purpose of the symptom is necessary. Another common example is a patient who asks for advice about a specific situation, but the therapist believes that his or her role should be limited to facilitating the patient in accepting responsibility for a course of action. The alternatives for dealing with these sorts of disagreements are either negotiation and compromise or dissolution of the therapeutic relationship (or at least, dissolution of the therapeutic alliance).

Negative Chemistry

Whatever the contributing factors, sometimes there is an unexplainable negative "chemistry," a spontaneous dislike of one party for the other, or both for each other. If the causes of this dislike are not discovered rapidly or some sort of accommodation made that alters these sentiments, then the relationship will, or should, end. If the patient does not abruptly terminate, the therapist has the opportunity to refer the patient to another clinician.

Transference–Countertransference Patterns

If the enactment of identifiable maladaptive patterns originating with the patient and usually ensnaring the therapist—that is, transference–countertransference patterns—reach a critical threshold of influence, they will interfere with the development and/or maintenance of a therapeutic alliance. At the same time, these interpersonal patterns often represent variations of the interpersonal problems that are the focus of therapeutic work. Therefore, they may represent a potentially invaluable opportunity for working with an active representation of a central problem.

Sometimes, a transference–countertransference enactment takes the form of a disagreement about therapeutic goals and/or tasks. For example, a 19-year-old woman was required to seek therapy by the court as part of her sentence for a crime for which she could have been incarcerated. She wanted her therapist to collude with her wish to merely show up for therapy appointments without engaging in meaningful work while telling the court that she was "in therapy." This situation paralleled the type of relationship that she demanded of her mother: to support her no matter what she did, because that was a mother's obligation to her child. This young woman's mother had doted on her throughout the patient's childhood, as a means of coping with a miserable marriage. When the mother finally divorced and found a more satisfying relationship, she abruptly ceased doting on her daughter, who was a young adolescent by then. The daughter responded with rage as well as self-destructive and socially disruptive acting-out behavior. When the therapist declined to be recruited into the desired parental role, the patient refused to discuss the situation and the relationship ended.

Temporal Constraints

The duration of therapy is all too often determined by factors other than the wishes of the participants. Such factors include the limits set by managed care policies, administrative policies of a clinic, or extraneous factors in the lives of the patient or the therapist. In such circumstances there may not be sufficient time for even basic therapeutic goals to be met. In this case, time, or the lack of it, operates as an obstacle to change.

The therapist's mental working models of personality and psychopathology guide him or her in constructing a cognitive map of portions of the patient's life relevant to the problems that are the focus of therapy. The cognitive map then guides the therapist in exploring this terrain. Likewise, the therapist's mental working model of therapeutic process guides his or her therapeutic interaction with the patient. Before attempting to change things, the therapist must first develop some knowledge of the patient and the problems to be addressed. This knowledge leads to the formulation of a central issue that serves as the focus of time-limited therapy. The process of developing a case formulation is the second competency and is the topic of Chapter 3.

NOTES

1. These developmental processes are detailed in the theoretical, clinical, and empirical literatures on "attachment theory" (e.g., Bowlby, 1969; Stern, 1985).

2. Earlier Strupp and I (Strupp & Binder, 1984) articulated a maladaptive version of this cyclical interpersonal process in our case formulation model, the cyclical maladaptive pattern (CMP). I will discuss the CMP in Chapter 3.

3. Alliance ruptures are synonymous with transference enactments (Safran & Muran, 2000). Many psychodynamically oriented therapists who conduct time-limited treatments assume that the patient's salient conflict will be enacted in the therapeutic relationship (i.e., as transference; Davanloo, 1980; Malan, 1976a; Safran & Muran, 2000; Strupp & Binder, 1984). In recent years, some brief dynamic therapists have suggested that such enactment is not inevitable, because there is not always sufficient time for this particular transference pattern to develop (e.g., Gustafson, 1995). In their study of Core Conflict Relationship Themes in relatively time-limited treatments, Connolly et al. (1996) found thematic parallels between outside relationships and the therapeutic relationship evident in some of their subjects but not in others. In other words, some patients did not evidence the salient interpersonal patterns identified outside of therapy, which were the foci of their treatments, in their relationships with their therapists. The role of transference in time-limited therapy is discussed in more detail in Chapter 5.

4. Monitoring the effectiveness of the therapeutic dialogue can be accomplished, session by session, with the use of various therapeutic process and outcome measures. For example, measures of the therapeutic alliance can be obtained from the patient after each session. Similarly, self-report measures of symptom levels and behavioral functioning can be obtained after each session. There is some evidence that feedback about the patient's status can be especially helpful when things are not going well (Lambert et al., 2002).

5. As I have argued, however, the essence of psychopathology represents the antithesis of this ability, namely interpersonal rigidity and stereotypy.

3

Competency 2

Problem Formulation and Treatment Planning

GENERAL ASSESSMENT ISSUES

In the first couple of meetings with a prospective patient, the therapist must make decisions about the nature of the individual's problems and whether or not psychotherapy appears to be the most appropriate type of intervention. Regardless of the intervention approach chosen, a preliminary strategy for implementing it and for gaining the patient's cooperation also must be developed. The knowledge and skills associated with implementing these assessment tasks constitute the second therapist competency.

At the beginning of an interview with someone who is seeking psychotherapy, the therapist is engaged in two parallel diagnostic tasks. One task involves developing an estimate about the degree and quality of psychological disturbance from which the patient suffers. This estimate can be codified with various nosological systems. For example, DSM-IV-TR (American Psychiatric Association, 2000) is a descriptive system of categorizing psychopathology in which clusters of behavioral and/or reportable signs and symptoms are distinguished. Another example, from psychoanalytic theory, is Kernberg's (1984) nosological system of categorizing psychopathology in terms of inferred levels of personality organization. These sorts of categorical systems provide a conceptual structure for estimating a patient's general

level of functioning and for determining whether or not psychotherapy is a viable form of intervention. These systems, however, are composed of categories that are too broad and/or abstract to guide the content of therapeutic interventions for any given patient. Gaining this
specificity is the function of the second diagnostic task: to develop a
formulation of the problem situation that is unique for this particular
patient at this point in his or her life. The content of such a formulation
should be sufficiently specific to guide the therapist's interventions.

The former diagnostic task can be called "descriptive diagnosis"
and the latter can be called "interpersonal diagnosis." Both tasks are
implemented, in unison, during the early part of the first interview, as
the clinician begins to form a preliminary impression about the patient's general level of disturbance. If the disturbance appears to be so
severe that interventions other than psychotherapy, or in addition to
psychotherapy, are required (e.g., immediate medication evaluation,
hospitalization, etc.), then the clinician's diagnostic efforts shift toward
completing a more thorough descriptive diagnosis, involving a more
structured review of the patient's mental status and current and past
areas of life functioning. If the patient's level of functioning appears to
be sufficient to allow him or her to maintain daily activities autono-
mously, and psychotherapy is indicated as the primary intervention,
then the clinician's diagnostic efforts shift toward completing a more
thorough interpersonal diagnosis, culminating in a content focus for
the therapy that is articulated in collaboration with the patient.

In the first two or three sessions of a therapy process, the therapist
may be relatively more structured in gathering pertinent information
for diagnostic and prognostic purposes than in subsequent sessions.
During this period, it is particularly important for the therapist to
maintain a balance between encouraging the patient to tell his or her
own story in his or her own terms and structuring the gathering of information in several crucial areas. An imbalance in either direction
may reduce the efficiency and effectiveness of the initial diagnostic
process. If the therapist only conducts a structured review of content
areas typically evaluated during a diagnostic evaluation, then he or
she may miss the patient's distinctive view of his or her problems and
characteristic style of conveying personal experiences. Furthermore,
the therapist may inadvertently induct the patient into a passive role
that significantly reduces the efficiency with which they can work
together—*and* is difficult to undo. On the other hand, if the therapist
only encourages the patient to spontaneously describe his or her life
and problems, without any direction, the therapist may not be able to

construct a coherent picture of those aspects of the patient's life that are relevant to the task of identifying a circumscribed set of problems.

Most books on time-limited psychotherapy emphasize evaluating areas of the patient's life that are relevant to an "interpersonal diagnosis" (e.g., Levenson, 1995; Magnavita, 1997). These areas include:

- The nature of the presenting problems, including the degree of distress, conflict, and impairment associated with these problems.
- The history of the presenting problems, including previous episodes.
- A cross-sectional examination of current activities, functioning, and life circumstances, and any significant variations in these areas over time.
- A cross-sectional examination of current relationships, and a history of significant work relationships, friendships, as well as romantic and other intimate relationships.
- An examination of family-of-origin relationships as well as family roles and dynamics.
- A family history of major physical and/or mental illnesses.
- An examination of any extraordinary events, such as losses, illnesses, financial setbacks, etc.
- An examination of any significant current or past emotional stressors, whether discrete or chronic.
- Any significant medical problems and/or prescription or nonprescription substance use.
- History of previous mental health treatment.
- Patient expectations about how treatment will be conducted and his or her goals.
- The nature of the unfolding therapeutic relationship that may reveal, in the form of transference–countertransference patterns, interpersonal manifestations of the problems to be addressed in therapy.
- Appraisal of the patient's reactions to "trial interventions," in order to gauge his or her spontaneous receptivity to the tasks required of the treatment model (i.e., the patient's readiness to form a working alliance).

The amount of attention devoted to any of these topics varies across patients and across topics at any given period during the course of a given therapy.

An additional factor that has received recent empirical support for its relationship to the development of a strong therapeutic alliance (Connolly-Gibbons et al., 2003) is the patient's expectations of improvement in therapy. This expectation probably reflects the patient's degree of trust in the potential benefits of human relations and therefore is a facet of his or her interpersonal relating style. It is a good idea to inquire about this issue on a routine basis. Any expression of pessimism, for example, should be addressed immediately.

WHO CAN BENEFIT FROM TIME-LIMITED THERAPY?

Clinical assessment has three broad aims. First, the clinician must gauge the overall quality and severity of the patient's psychopathology. This judgment is most often codified with DSM-IV multiaxial descriptors (American Psychiatric Association, 2000). Second, the clinician must decide upon an intervention strategy. In addition to psychotherapy, such strategies include pharmacotherapy, inpatient milieu treatment, intervention with others in the person's social network, and assistance from social agencies in managing practical problems, to name a few common alternatives and/or adjuncts. If psychotherapy is the chosen strategy, a problem formulation must be developed to guide the type and content of therapeutic interventions. Third, the clinician must begin to develop a therapeutic alliance with the patient, as a foundation for whatever collaborative work is mutually undertaken.

The early pioneers of time-limited dynamic therapy only partially broke free of the technical assumptions associated with traditional open-ended psychoanalytic therapy. Although they boldly innovated brief treatment approaches, they still held attitudes associated with a long-term treatment perspective. One of these attitudes was that the relatively short duration of brief therapy severely constrains the variety of patients for whom the treatment is suitable. It was assumed that a thorough, detailed assessment must be conducted in order to identify those patients who have the necessary "ego strengths" to engage in the specific tasks required of the given therapy approach. Suitable patients were thought to be those with relatively circumscribed psychopathology and demonstrably high functioning (e.g., Davanloo, 1980; Malan, 1976a; Mann, 1973; Sifneos, 1979). Contemporary practitioners of dynamic time-limited treatments tend to have more liberal attitudes about the range of treatable problems and persons, although extensive assessment efforts are still recommended to optimize patient selection and treatment planning (e.g., Della Selva, 1996; Magnavita, 1997; Zois & Scarpa, 1997).

In contrast, the experiences of other veteran clinical researchers and teachers have led to the alternative view that most patients for whom psychotherapy is an appropriate intervention can be helped by a time-limited approach, and such patients can be identified without an extensive and structured formal evaluation (e.g., Garfield, 1998; Wolberg, 1980). For example, the venerable clinician/teacher Lewis Wolberg put it this way: "The best strategy, in my opinion, is to assume that every patient, irrespective of diagnosis, will respond to short-term treatment unless he proves himself refractory to it" (Wolberg, 1980, p. 140). In a similar vein, Garfield has stated that "brief therapy can be considered for most patients who are in touch with reality, are experiencing some discomfort, and have made the effort to seek help for their difficulties" (1998, p. 21). The kinds of problems that might be considered unsuitable for an outpatient psychotherapeutic intervention would include psychotic disorganization, chronic incoherence, socially disruptive impulsivity, and perhaps active suicidal and/or homicidal urges. However, a pharmacotherapeutic intervention and possibly a concurrent temporary hospitalization or other intensive interventions, with the aid of community resources, might reduce these sorts of symptoms to a level that is manageable in brief psychotherapy. On the other hand, character traits that indicate a severely damaged personality—such as dishonesty, a lack of concern for, and integrity in, human relationships, and no motivation to take responsibility for problems—almost always indicate that the individual will not benefit from psychotherapy. Unfortunately, medications and other treatment approaches are not likely to render a person with these personality traits any more amenable to psychotherapeutic influence (Gustafson, 1995).

Within the parameters bounded by these extreme sorts of symptomatic and character pathologies, relevant empirical research supports a very flexible approach to treatment selection criteria. On the whole, pretherapy patient characteristics (including diagnosis, most personality characteristics, adjustment, and demographic variables) are not significantly predictive of psychotherapy outcome (Binder et al., 1987; Garfield, 1994).[1] Dose–effect research over the past 15 years, however, indicates that the greater the severity of a patient's psychopathology, the slower will be his or her response to treatment and the more treatment sessions will be needed to produce clinically significant change (Kopta et al., 1994; Lambert, Hansen, & Finch, 2001).

There does appear to be a strong relationship, however, between one personality variable and treatment outcome. This variable is "quality of interpersonal relating," defined in terms of relative levels of maturity (Hoglend, Sorlie, Heyerdahl, Sorbye, & Amlo, 1993; Piper, Joyce, McCallum, & Azim, 1998). A developmentally immature level of interpersonal relating includes characteristics such as experiencing personal needs as peremptory, manipulating others without regard to their feelings, inability to tolerate interpersonal separations or losses, insensitivity to interpersonal boundaries, exquisite sensitivities to slights and criticism, primarily hostile or cool mood states, and difficulty with self-reflection and accepting personal responsibility for one's actions. In contrast, a more developmentally mature level of relating includes characteristics such as the capacity to empathize with the personal experiences of another, the capacity to tolerate being independent or alone, the ability to balance emotional intimacy with respect for interpersonal boundaries, mood states that include the potential for periods of warmth and humor, and at least the potential for self-reflection and self-responsibility.

Although research instruments and protocols exist for reliably assessing quality of interpersonal relating, these methods have not been adapted for use in everyday practice (e.g., Piper & Duncan, 1999). Consequently, there are no clear, practical criteria and procedures for the practitioner to use to reliably and validly assess quality of interpersonal relating. Some helpful questions the clinician can ask him- or herself in making this assessment include the following:

1. Does it appear that we can reach an agreement on goals and methods of working together?
2. Based on this person's communications, can I construct a clear and coherent mental picture of his or her interpersonal relationships, both present and past?
3. Is this person curious about him- or herself?
4. Does this person accept responsibility for his or her contributions to the problems?
5. Does this person appear to be open to new ideas that I might introduce?
6. Does this person describe his or her problems in interpersonal terms?

Another method of assessing the level of a patient's maturity in interpersonal relating is by examining the therapist's personal reaction to the patient. This subjective experience, defined broadly as a form of countertransference (Levenson, 1995; Strupp & Binder, 1984), can be an important factor in gauging the potential for a prospective patient and therapist to establish a productive and collaborative working relationship. Sustained negative reactions on the part of the therapist, regardless of how subtle or fleeting, usually signal a serious defect in the patient's ability to relate in the sort of intimate and collaborative way that is crucial for significant therapeutic work to be accomplished. For example, a businessman in his late 40s made an appointment with an experienced male therapist. The patient had been married for over 25 years and had several adult children who were out of the house or almost ready to leave. He cited chronic marital problems as the reason he had contacted the therapist. At the same time, the patient related to the therapist in a challenging and dismissive manner, conveying the attitude, in word and tone, that the patient had no interest in anything the therapist had to say. The therapist, in turn, felt an instant dislike for the patient. It turned out that the patient had made the appointment in response to an ultimatum from his wife: either talk to a therapist about his treatment of her, about which she felt miserable, or she would leave him. The patient stated that he did not love his wife, saw no future in the relationship, and probably never should have married her. Yet he did not reveal these sentiments to his wife, nor did he make any attempt to end the marriage. Although the patient appeared more ambivalent about ending his marriage than he acknowledged, he emphatically stated that he had no problems nor any interest in considering his behavior in the marriage. When the first appointment ended, neither party had any desire to meet again.

On the other hand, the therapist may have an initially negative reaction to a new patient that shifts toward more positive sentiments as subsequent contact provides greater understanding—which is conveyed to the patient, who, in turn, shows appreciation for this interest. For example, a woman in her middle 50s who suffered from chronic depression was referred by her psychiatrist to a psychotherapist. She was in her second unhappy marriage. Her first marriage, which had lasted over 10 years, was disappointing because she found her husband to be very controlling and "stodgy." Her second marriage, lasting over 20 years, was even more disappointing because her husband was irresponsible and childish. At first contact, the patient's male therapist felt an instant dislike for the patient. In his mind he immediately labeled her as passive–aggressive, a term he knew was as much pejorative as informing. His response came on the heels of her complaints about the therapist's office location, the parking situation, and the layout, all of which were voiced on the way from the waiting room to the office (e.g., "This step is hard to see. It would be easy for someone to stumble over it and hurt themselves."). Once seated, the patient began to tell her story. Since childhood, her role in significant relationships had been to "clean up other peoples' messes," for which she received no acknowledgment. She had spent her life futilely yearning for someone upon whom she could lean and with whom she would feel supported and safe. As the therapist comprehended this lifelong theme, he conveyed his understanding to her and felt more compassionate toward her. She, in turn, became tearful and expressed her appreciation of the therapist's understanding, which she had not previously experienced with anyone else. After a shaky start, they were able to establish a strong therapeutic alliance.

The same body of research that has found a relationship between quality of interpersonal relating and treatment outcome has also identified an important mediating variable that has implications for treatment planning. The patient's level of maturity in interpersonal relating appears to contribute to determining the kind of working relationship established with the therapist (i.e., in the therapeutic alliance) that will be most effective in producing a positive therapeutic outcome (Connolly-Gibbons et al., 2003; Hoglend et al., 1993; Piper et al., 1993; Piper et al., 1998). This research has supported and given enhanced conceptual precision to a therapeutic principle proposed by Luborsky (1984): the patient's quality of interpersonal relating dictates his or her spontaneous ability to remain committed to the therapeutic work even while being confronted with uncomfortable issues. The less mature or competent the patient is in interpersonal relating, the more the therapist must actively nurture and support the patient's continued involvement in the therapeutic relationship.

Time-limited treatment models "factor in" the patient's capacity for involvement in the therapeutic relationship and the tasks of therapy. For example, Malan (1976a), Davanloo (1980), and Sifneos (1979) purposefully developed their models with patients who possessed relatively high levels of interpersonal relating. Consequently, the strategy characterizing these models involves aggressive confrontation of identified problems and reliance on patients' innate capacity for interpersonal engagement to support the therapeutic alliance. In contrast, treatment models developed with patients who were more likely to evidence immaturity in their interpersonal relating are characterized by a strategy that places relatively more emphasis on nurturing the therapeutic alliance and identifying and repairing breaches in it (Levenson, 1995; Safran & Muran, 2000; Strupp & Binder, 1984; Seruya, 1997). Still other approaches, directly following Luborsky's (1984) recommendation, attempt to implement either an "expressive" or a "supportive" therapeutic strategy, based on a clinical judgment about the patient's quality of interpersonal relating (during the course of therapy the therapist may shift this strategy in response to the changing state of the therapeutic alliance; Book, 1998; Magnavita, 1997).

DIAGNOSTIC INQUIRY SHOULD BE THERAPEUTIC: PRELIMINARY EXPLORATION

The initial contact with a new patient involves "reconnaissance" (Sullivan, 1954), as the therapist feels his or her way in the new relationship. Anticipating the first interview with a new patient may evoke feelings that are similar to those experienced when meeting anyone new: a combination of curiosity, excitement, and possibly apprehension. Even though a therapist has a particular job to do, the task must be performed initially in a new relationship, and entering this relationship is like beginning a journey into unfamiliar territory. The therapist attempts to get to know the other person and simultaneously to nurture the embryonic relationship, because anything done together will be more satisfying and productive and contribute to the creation of a solid interpersonal foundation (Horvath & Greenberg, 1994). Because the nascent therapeutic relationship has some fundamental aspects in common with any new human relationship, the novice therapist can compensate for a lack of professional experience, to some extent, by drawing on his or her personal experiences for guidance. The seasoned therapist has the advantage of being able to draw upon both personal and professional experiences to guide him or her in this new relationship. Competent and expert practitioners use analogical reasoning when they face new situations; that is, their ability to understand and act in a new situation is enhanced by their ability to perceive relevant similarities between this new situation and prior situations with which they have dealt (Sternberg, 1977).

The two major purposes of clinical assessment are (1) to construct a clear picture of a person's distress, dissatisfaction, or psychological dysfunctioning, and (2) to generate a set of questions and hypotheses about why this state of affairs exists. The early pioneers of short-term dynamic therapies advocated conducting exhaustive evaluation efforts that often were impractical outside of a research and/or training institution. In contrast, the time constraints imposed by current health care policymakers have pushed many short-term therapists into making rapid interventions, with little or no time devoted to identifying or understanding the problems to be addressed. Therapists who proceed in this way attempt to implement treatment as a solution to problems *before they fully understand those problems.* A hallmark of an expert in any profession is the time devoted to gaining a thorough understanding of a problem before initiating extensive action. In contrast, novices (or those who act like novices) tend to plunge into action with trial-and-error strategies (Glaser & Chi, 1988). A patient may initially divulge an overwhelming amount of information or present a bewildering account of longstanding unhappiness. Trying to help this patient without a conceptual blueprint of the problem area to guide interventions is likely to be inefficient and ineffective. Of course, developing a coherent diagnostic picture is not easy. The very concept of "psychopathology" rests upon hypothetical constructs (e.g., "major depressive disorder," "borderline personality disorder") involving arbitrary conceptual boundaries that are recurrently modified and which fit no individual exactly. Individualized, theory-guided problem formulations are more useful for guiding therapeutic interventions but take a great deal of skill to keep in sight.The ill-defined nature of psychopathology makes it all the more important for therapists to conduct a thorough analysis of the problem context, in order to establish workable boundaries around the problem (i.e., a therapeutic focus).

Another reason for clarifying a patient's problems: The precision with which therapeutic goals can be defined is largely a function of how precisely the problems have been defined. For example, if the problem is defined as "low self-esteem," the corollary therapeutic goal would be to raise the patient's self-esteem to a "healthy" level. But how does the therapist precisely determine when the patient's self-esteem has reached this level? In contrast, the self-esteem problem can be defined more precisely in loosely behavioral and cognitive terms: The patient strives to please other people, even if it means sacrificing her own needs, because she is convinced that she is not worthy of the regard of others. The therapeutic goal that is the corollary to this problem formulation would be one in which the patient demonstrates an ability to relate with others in a way that meets the needs of both, because he or she feels worthy of this sort of reciprocal relationship.

A distinction should be made between these patient-specific treatment goals and the relatively more generic goals involving the acquisition or refinement of practice skills such as self-monitoring and reflection-in-action. A therapist encourages the achievement of a generic goal such as reflection-in-action, for example, when he or she encourages the patient to catch him- or herself, between sessions enacting an identified maladaptive scenario, and to question the previously unquestioned assumptions about self and others that are driving the patient's behavior in the scenario. The achievement of these generic goals enables the person to identify and manage future problems. Both types of goals (i.e., patient-specific and generic) should be part of every psychotherapy case formulation.

Devoting attention to careful diagnostic evaluation does not preclude rapidly intervening to help patients in distress. In fact, the process of gaining an understanding of a patient's problems overlaps the efforts at resolving these problems (Strupp & Binder, 1984). In psychotherapy, diagnostic and intervention activities should always proceed simultaneously; more experienced and proficient therapists will be able to achieve these twin aims with particular efficiency. Whereas experts devote more attention than novices to understanding a problem, they also are quicker to form an effective working model of the problem and to begin intervening, because they are more efficient at identifying and organizing relevant information (Chi et al., 1988; Sandifer, Hordern, & Green, 1970).

The process by which diagnostic understanding and therapeutic intervention proceed in interrelated fashion is one instance of a generic problem-solving process called "reflective conversations" (Schon, 1983, 1987). The practitioner in any performance domain is continually on alert to receive feedback from the problem situation about the consequences of his or her interventions. This feedback modifies and enhances the practitioner's understanding of the problem situation and points to new interventions. To paraphrase Schon: *The problem situation is changed in the process of understanding it, and it is understood in the process of changing it*. In the psychotherapy setting the reflective conversation is usually a dialogue with a person, the patient. Furthermore, the diagnostic and intervention facets of a therapeutic inquiry are often indistinguishable. For example, in order to gain additional information, the clinician asks the patient a trenchant question about some facet of his or her problem. Not only does the patient's answer potentially aid the diagnostic task by providing informative content, but in the act of formulating an answer the patient may be stimulated to think, perceive, or reflect in new ways upon an old problem. In this way, a therapeutic process is facilitated. Below is an example of diagnostic and therapeutic processes operating simultaneously as the therapist has a reflective conversation with the patient.

Carl is a man in his early 30s who is married and has a little boy. He described his marriage as lacking emotional intimacy, about which his wife repeatedly complains. Carl described the reason for seeking therapy in the following way:

P: I am not as satisfied with my life as I think I should be. My relationships with people are not as fulfilling as I would like; they don't seem as satisfying as they should be. This is true with my wife and child, and I am not happy about this. In a lot of ways, my wife and I can deal with this, but it just isn't working right. I also have a hard time in social situations making friends. I really don't have any close friends.

In general terms, Carl describes an unpleasant emotional barrier between himself and others. The therapist asks for a specific, concrete example. This is the most effective strategy for constructing a vivid and precise mental picture (i.e., working model) of the patient's problem.

T: Can you give me an example of when you have a hard time in social situations with people?

P: Well, recently I decided to join a musical group that performs for social functions at our church. I enjoy playing the piano. I thought it might be a good way to get involved with a small group of people with common interests. I did meet one person, but the other people ignored me. I didn't feel that I fit in. The person I met talked to me and encouraged me to come back. I really felt uncomfortable and came out feeling that I had not really made any contacts there.

Carl goes on to describe feeling "stifled" while he was at the meeting. The therapist inquires about the meaning of this term.

T: Stifled?

P: Sort of. But *stifled* implies that something outside me is doing it, which I don't feel.

T: Well, stifled . . . you were somehow stifling yourself, drawing back
   from the others.

This brief give-and-take clarifies that Carl stifles his spontaneity in
certain interpersonal situations, which may contribute to the emotional
barrier about which he complains.

P: I don't believe that anyone there was stifling me, but I am not
   aware of doing it to myself. It took a real effort to go to that meeting. I am glad that I went and plan to go back. I really hope that I
   will get to know some people there.

The therapist continues to direct the diagnostic inquiry toward
specific illustrations of Carl's problem.

T: You mentioned that you didn't feel that you "fit in." Can you elaborate on that experience a little more?

P: Well, I arrived a little late, and the group was already playing, and
   they sounded really good. They sounded like they had played together for a long time—but I have not played in groups very much.
   Between songs the group leader asked me to join them, but I told
   him I wasn't really sure I was going to perform with them. Maybe I
   will just rehearse with them but not actually perform. He said I
   should stick around and see how I liked it. I told him I wasn't sure
   how much the group would like my playing.

T: You describe how you felt like you didn't fit in, at least in one
   sense, in terms of not knowing whether or not you'd measure up to
   their expectations.

Based on what Carl had recalled so far about his experience with
the musical group, the therapist had formed an initial diagnostic hypothesis that Carl's interpersonal discomfort was caused by a sense of
inferiority. Specifically, the therapist hypothesized that Carl was afraid
that others would criticize his performance in certain interpersonal situations. This is a plausible hypothesis and a very common source of
interpersonal discomfort and inhibition. As we shall see, however, it is
not the primary source of this patient's discomfort.

P: That was a big part of it. I was very conscious of it, but there is
   something more than that which is harder for me to put my finger
   on. I really don't know how to put this. I think I almost never feel

like I am part of a group. If I'm in a group, I usually feel like everyone else has reasons for being there that I don't have.

T: Because you don't measure up or some other reason?

Already the therapist begins to question his initial hypothesis
about the cause of Carl's discomfort, in response to the (reflective) conversation ensuing after he presented it. The patient spontaneously
shifts to a new example of a situation in which he experienced an emotional barrier.

P: Not necessarily that. In this case the expectation pressure was there,
and that was one thing I was really conscious of. In the company I
work for, I know that I do a good job and am a valued employee.
But I really don't feel that I have company loyalty, that the company's interests are the most important thing to me. They talk
about working as a team, and I imagine that the other employees
feel that they are working as a team united by the primary motive
of advancing the company. I have never felt that.

T: What do you feel instead?

P: Well, I feel that the people who run the company have the company's best interests at heart, but not necessarily *my* best interests. I
feel that if my primary interest was the good of the company, I
would be exploited somehow. Other employees don't seem to feel
this way.

T: So one example of feeling a part of a group is feeling like you're not
going to measure up to their standards of performance, and another one, if I'm hearing you right, regarding your work for this
company, is that you have different values and priorities from the
other people in the company. You just don't feel part of the spirit.

P: Right.

In this brief, early diagnostic interchange, the therapist fosters a
reflective conversation with his patient that produces a hypothesis
concerning the source of the patient's interpersonal discomfort and
inhibition. The dialogue quickly reveals, however, that this initial
hypothesis may be off the mark. Further inquiry suggests a new diagnostic hypothesis concerning motives for participating in group activities that Carl implies are selfish and that set him apart from those
around him. Carl says this issue is "harder to put my finger on." Clarifying his experience around this issue of motives that are hidden from

others involves his learning something new about himself. This sort of exploratory inquiry (i.e., reconnaissance) is a fundamental part of the therapeutic process and an example of the continuous intersection of diagnostic and therapeutic processes.

GUIDELINES FOR THE DIAGNOSTIC INQUIRY

The ultimate goal of a diagnostic inquiry is the construction of a case formulation that can effectively guide therapeutic interventions. The essence of a dynamic–interpersonal formulation is an interpersonal story line or subplot that represents an important and distressing issue at this point in the evolving narrative of the patient's life. From the first moment of a therapeutic encounter, the therapist's most useful mental resources for constructing a case formulation are *curiosity* and *common sense*.[2] Curiosity focuses the therapist's attention on what the patient is saying as well as on how he or she characteristically conveys information and relates to others. When there is any hint of ambiguity in the patient's communications, the curious therapist inquires about precise details and meanings. As a result, the therapist's mental working model of the patient and their therapeutic relationship is more precise and vivid, which, in turn, enables him or her to take more effective therapeutic actions. Curiosity also helps the therapist maintain his or her poise during interpersonally difficult (particularly hostile) encounters with a patient. Interpersonal tension or conflict can be particularly disconcerting in a new relationship, because the therapist knows so little about the patient. It can feel like being lost on a stormy night in an unfamiliar place. A curious therapist, however, can maintain emotional equilibrium with questions such as, "How did we get into this situation?", "Do the circumstances associated with this quandary provide any clues as to the nature of the patient's problem?", "What are we respectively contributing to this situation?"

Common sense leads a therapist to appraise the degree of fit between the patient's way of construing and conducting his or her life and what the therapist, representing a hypothetical consensus of reasonable persons, would consider to be reasonable and rational under the same circumstances. This mind-set, too, is especially useful for novice therapists who do not have extensive professional experiences and well integrated theoretical prescriptions upon which to draw, but who usually see relevant similarities between the patient's circumstances and their own prior personal experiences. Of course, a thera-

pist's use of his or her common sense to evaluate the behavior of a patient goes beyond an unwavering empathic stance. Although empathic
receptivity, per se, is a necessary therapeutic function, in most cases it
is not sufficient to conduce change. Any act initiated by the therapist
for the purpose of influencing the patient implies some sort of value
judgment. The therapist should not try to ignore or deny his or her values when working with a patient. Rather, the therapist attempts to remain continuously aware of what values he or she is conveying to the
patient. It is assumed that the therapist has a more constructive view of
those areas of life that are problematic for the patient and therefore is
able to identify discrepancies between his or her picture and the one
presented by the patient. These discrepancies, in turn, indicate topics
to pursue in therapy.[3]

An example of such a discrepancy in the picture of an interpersonal situation is found in the initial diagnostic interview with Carl,
who experienced an emotional barrier with other people. In response
to the therapist's encouragement, he elaborated on the first meeting
with his church musical group, which he had intended to join because
he enjoyed music and wanted to make friends. This was a situation,
however, where he felt out of place.

P: I know that I could have made more of an effort to reach out, but I
   don't want to seem overeager or assertive, or whatever. I just didn't
   feel like making that effort.

T: You didn't feel like doing that?

P: No, I didn't.

T: Do you have a sense of what stopped you?

P: Well, it seems like all I felt like saying were self-deprecating things
   about my musical ability. Also, everyone introduced themselves to
   me, but I couldn't remember their names.

T: Did it occur to you to, for instance, to approach people and ask
   them about what kind of music they like to play, about their performances, and what role you could play?

The point of this question was not to teach Carl social skills but to
elicit his reaction to a commonsense interpersonal strategy. This reaction might shed light on the internal working model that contributed
to his discomfort and inhibition in this situation.

P: We did talk about some of that and the next time the group would be meeting. As I was leaving, I was walking out with this guy who plays the guitar, which I also like, and I talked to him a little bit, and I told him I was going to learn my parts. We exchanged some pleasant words. His wife showed up, and she kind of joined in our conversation. People were sort of grouped in little groups of mostly two people talking together. The group is very small. I suppose there were 10 of us there, all together. Some left and about four others went outside and were talking, two and two, and then there was me and this guy, and there might have been a group of about two or three inside. It was hard to be a part of it. I don't know if that is just an excuse.

The therapist's curiosity about this interpersonal encounter helped him to form a clear mental picture of the scene described by the patient, and also helped him to notice a small discrepancy between this imagined scene and the patient's reported experience of feeling left out or out of place.

T: The picture I have is, OK, there's this small musical group. After it ended, people broke off into pairs and were talking to each other. Apparently, they knew each other. Yet you did the same thing. I mean, if people had come in off the street, they would have seen this small group, divided into pairs, and they would see you talking to this man, and then the man and his wife, as the other people also continued talking. And yet even though it sounds like you were doing the same thing everybody else was doing, you felt somehow not a part of it, ignored.

P: Good point. That's a good point.

In pointing out this discrepancy between the nature of the interpersonal situation and the patient's experience of it, the therapist incited the patient to take a closer look at his presumptions about such situations. This careful differentiation led to the discovery of a new facet of the patient's interpersonal discomfort and inhibition—and, ultimately, to a new hypothesis about the source of the problem.

The mind-sets of curiosity and common sense are generic interpersonal capacities; they help an individual navigate effectively in any interpersonal encounter or relationship. Novice therapists can use their own past interpersonal experiences as frames of reference for appraising the constructiveness and reasonableness of patients' ways of construing their interpersonal experiences and their styles of interpersonal relating. More experienced therapists have the additional benefit of their cumulative therapeutic experiences. The therapist can also use his or her common sense to construct hypothetical working models of healthy situations to mentally superimpose over the pictures constructed from the patient's descriptions of his or her life. Discrepancies between the therapist's prototypic healthy mental models and the mental models reflecting the patient's life point to interpersonal psychopathology.

Curiosity and common sense also help the therapist to generate *incisive questions* that are thematically relevant to the patient's main problems and to the immediate line of inquiry. Not only are they indispensable to the task of gathering relevant information for assessment (i.e., for articulating a problem), they also stimulate thinking about problems from new and creative perspectives. Furthermore, incisive questions incite the patient to take responsibility for his or her problems and to effectively contribute to their resolution.

Incisive questions can be very probing. The amount and depth of probing diagnostic inquiry that a patient can tolerate depends on several factors: (1) the patient's psychological mindedness, (2) tolerance for uncomfortable psychological experiences, (3) self-reflectiveness, and (4) trust in the therapist. Patients who have these characteristics are more likely to contribute to the formation of a strong therapeutic alliance. If the therapeutic alliance is relatively strong, the relationship can withstand a more probing and confrontative inquiry by the therapist; if the patient perceives the therapist as intrusive, the latter can always "back off." On the other hand, when the alliance is fragile, even apparently innocuous questions may be experienced as intrusive, threatening, or hostile. A patient may presume that the intentions behind the therapist's questions are malevolent or manipulative. With such a patient, the therapist should remain continually attentive to the his or her reactions to the inquiry. Flexibility enables the therapist to balance the probings of diagnostic inquiry with the supportive activities of maintaining a therapeutic alliance. How to approach a new patient in a way that encourages him or her to "open up" usually involves improvising in an unfamiliar situation. A therapist must rely on the interpersonal skills that have been acquired over a lifetime, both personal and professional. Novice therapists must be especially careful not to let their absorption in learning new therapy techniques overshadow the interpersonal skills that they already possess.

When obtaining historical information from the patient, it is prudent to keep in mind that the particulars conveyed are consciously selected, more or less, by the patient from a wealth of information that could be presented. The question then becomes, "Why is the patient telling me this information in this particular way?" From a relational perspective, the answer is that the patient is conveying, with varying degrees of deliberateness a "story" about his or her life as currently experienced. Consequently, the historical information conveyed may or may not be factual, but it assuredly reflects the patient's conscious and unconscious views of his or her life, including the experience of talking to a therapist. The content and quality of the information provided by the patient is determined by several factors, including (1) the particular story being told, as it reflects the patient's current conscious and unconscious experiences of his or her life; (2) the patient's storytelling style and ability; and (3) the nature of the evolving therapeutic relationship, particularly the kind of dialogue that is fostered by the therapist.

The relational perspective of "facts"—or their nonexistence— reflects a constructivist theory of knowledge (i.e., an epistemology; Neimeyer & Mahoney, 1995) in which objective reality is not capable of being objectively "discovered"; rather, each human mind actively— albeit, tacitly—constructs its own unique organization of its perception of the surrounding world. Specifically, the human mind organizes and structures experience in order to give it *meaning*. Interpersonal meanings are organized in the form of a narration, which provides meaningful sequences of action and transaction. From the recurrent narrations of an individual can be culled meaningful patterns of interaction that characterize that person's interpersonal relationships. This view of interpersonal experience has an important implication for the role of psychotherapy. The individual is seen as both the author of as well as an actor in his or her recurrent interpersonal scenarios. In other words, even if the individual feels like a helpless victim of his or her fate, usually he or she actively and unwittingly participates in self-defeating perpetuation of the interpersonal drama (Hoffman, 1983; Lyddon, 1995; Neimeyer, 1997a, 1997b).

From a relational–constructivist perspective, psychotherapy is essentially a collaborative process of constructing and reconstructing meaningful interpersonal narratives. The therapist may aim interventions directly at modifying symptoms or at modifying the interpersonal story that is seen as contributing to the production of symptoms. The initial construction of a salient interpersonal narrative serves as the context for the patient's presenting problems. Whatever historical and current information is communicated, as well as the manner in which it is conveyed, contains salient interpersonal themes around which the patient's personality is currently organized. The patient's recalled history is relevant and therapeutic to the extent that it provides a meaningful hypothetical origin for the patient's current dysfunctional mental activity and maladaptive interpersonal interactions. Santayana (1905) warned that those who cannot remember the past are doomed to repeat it. The past does not, however, have to be represented by relics of veridical facts. From a constructivist perspective, the retrospective creation of a currently influential narrative theme can represent the past. Pointing out to patients that the currently constructed interpersonal context occurred in the past but that they are coping with their life as it is now can often encourage them to break ingrained maladaptive patterns of experiencing and acting. It dawns on patients that circumstances are now very different. Whether constructing a meaningful hypothetical past or a current interpersonal reality, the following criteria for gauging the adequacy of the construction can be applied:

1. Does it provide a plausible organization of the available information?
2. Does it provide a narrative theme that resonates meaningfully with the patient's experience?
3. Does it potentially promote a sense of agency and participation in the patient?
4. Does it offer the potential for discovering alternative versions of what, up to this point, has been assumed to be unequivocally "true"?

In the psychoanalytic theory of therapy, hypothetical reconstructions of past events for the purpose of making sense of unconscious motivations for present behavior are called "reconstructive interpretations" (Greenson, 1967). An example of such a hypothetical reconstruction occurred several sessions into Carl's treatment. During this session, Carl and his therapist had identified a link between Carl's expectation that his desire for emotionally close relationships with others would be rebuffed and his childhood relationship with his emotionally constricted and aloof father.

P: I think both in his actions and his reactions, my father doesn't tell you about things that he is uncomfortable with. On the contrary, he'll withdraw if he's uncomfortable. And in his reactions, if he senses that you are coming to him with something that you're uncomfortable with, he'll also withdraw. I guess that I picked up from those behaviors that that is the way to behave, both because it's a good way to get along with him, and also because that's the way he behaves.

T: I was wondering about that, too. It sounded a lot like the way you described your father and your relationship with him. It makes me wonder if the way you experienced your relationship with him— the way you interpreted his emotional distance—is the prototype for other relationships. Maybe he is not interested in you or doesn't even like you. By not even liking you, I mean, look, you're growing up, you're a little kid, and here you have this imposing figure, your father. You're bursting with all kinds of things that you want to tell him, reactions that you want from him. And he doesn't seem to want to listen to you or give anything back. What conclusion can you draw? The obvious conclusion a kid would draw is that he doesn't want to be bothered with you, doesn't even like you. You're not worth the bother. What I'm suggesting is more than just speculation, because look at what you experienced with me today. You have described me as "reserved," and that must mean that I don't want to be bothered by your feelings, and maybe I don't even like you.

The hypothetical childhood scenario depicted by Carl's therapist may never have occurred, but it captured a narrative meaning that resonated with Carl's sense of his childhood relationship with his father and with his current experience of relationships. In this particular example, the therapist was able to reinforce the relevance of the hypothetical scenario by linking it forward to how Carl had been construing their relationship. A major indication of the relevance and good timing of an interpretive intervention is that it spurs a productive therapeutic inquiry. In this case, Carl became more aware of how much he missed not having a closer relationship with his father.

During this work, the therapist pointed out how Carl simultaneously described feeling sad about the absence of a closer relationship with his father, while he automatically stifled the experience of this feeling in the presence of his male therapist. The therapist suggested that Carl was creating an emotional barrier between himself and his therapist, because he assumed that, like his father, his therapist would be acutely uncomfortable with Carl's feelings and would withdraw. This observation had a deep impact on Carl, who commented on the irrationality of his current behavior. His therapist responded with another hypothetical reconstruction of Carl's childhood relationship with his father, to demonstrate that in light of his history, Carl's present way of relating to significant others had a purpose.

T: You know, in the context of what we're talking about—how you experience your father—your behavior with me is not irrational at all. It seems so reasonable, especially if you decided, as a young boy that your father did not want to be burdened with your feelings, with your needs for closeness, with your feelings whatever they were. You obviously wanted his approval; you wanted to be loved by him, not rejected. What else could you do? The more you wanted to be closer, the more you wanted to share, the more you had to stifle all that you wanted, because you felt that he wanted you to keep to yourself. Just like, again, earlier today, you said you were going to hold back and wait and see what I will approve of, what I will sanction. And if I don't give it to you in writing, then you decide that I won't sanction anything.

P: Right now, all I can say is that I believe that it makes sense to me.

In Carl's therapy, the therapist was able to identify and use transference enactments of his central issue around constructing emotional barriers, in this case with his therapist. Many time-limited psychodynamic therapists assume that the patient's experience of, and actions in, the evolving therapeutic relationship always contain the most immediate version of his or her central issue, and, as such, should always be the focus of inquiry (Davanloo, 1980; Levenson, 1995; Malan, 1976a; Strupp & Binder, 1984). However, this common working assumption does not apply in many, if not most, brief therapies conducted today. Rather, the most promising area of the patient's life in which to search for a central issue is his or her current relationships.[4] Nevertheless, it is good practice to always remain alert to evidence of a patient's central issue being enacted within the therapeutic relationship in the form of transference and to pursue exploration of this interpersonal pattern, if the patient is willing.

THE PROBLEM FORMULATION MODEL:
CYCLICAL MALADAPTIVE PATTERN

People who can benefit from psychotherapy typically present a conglomeration of symptoms, character foibles, and relationship problems. In order to formulate an interpersonal diagnosis, the therapist needs an organizing principle to guide the selection, organization, and prioritization of clinical data into a coherent picture of a circumscribed problem. The nature of this problem, in turn, guides the formulation of goals and intervention strategies. Without a conceptual map of the problem context to provide direction, interventions are more liable to be irrelevant or ineffective. The therapist would be navigating in the dark, without guiding indicators. An interpersonal diagnosis involves identifying a central issue that underlies the patient's presenting problems (or "disorder") and that can be traced back through his or her personal history (Eells, 1997; Messer & Wolitzky, 1997; Strupp & Binder, 1984). The identification of a therapeutic focus fosters the "selective attention" (Balint, Ornstein, & Balint, 1972) required to efficiently filter the profuse clinical data produced in a therapeutic encounter. Precisely describing a therapeutic focus is comparable to increasing the resolution of a microscope; it enhances the clarity and detail of the objects (in this case, psychological problems) that are being observed.

From a dynamic–interpersonal theoretical perspective, the problem formulation is constructed in the form of a "narrative structure," in which experiences and actions are sequentially organized into predictable patterns of interpersonal experiencing and acting (Messer & Wolitsky, 1997). A narrative structure is part of a life story composed of one or a few central, organizing interpersonal themes. These themes provide a "coherent, comprehensive, plausible, and reasonably accurate account" (Strupp & Binder, 1984, p. 33) of the facets of an individual's personality development and current functioning that is relevant to the psychological problems to be addressed. A case formulation constructed as part of a life story represents a diagnosis that is precisely individualized for each patient. The story uniquely associated with a patient should explain the source of interpersonal problems as well as help explain his or her distressing symptoms and impairments in functioning. By contrast, a descriptive psychopathology diagnosis represents an abstract category that only describes a prototypic syndrome of signs, symptoms, and traits that any given person will only approximate.

As therapist and patient construct an interpersonal theme that gives narrative coherence to that facet of the patient's life that has been associated with his or her problems, the patient has the opportunity to realize that an interpersonal theme, regardless of how influential, is potentially *alterable*. As an unconscious influence, an interpersonal theme can have the aura of indisputable reality. As a conscious story line, interpersonal themes make the patient's self-defeating and confusing actions and experiences intelligible. At the same time, the patient can appreciate that his or her story is merely one version of reality, and other versions are more possible than they had ever imagined (Schacht et al., 1984).

The particular narrative structure that characterizes the formulation model describes human actions embedded in the context of interpersonal transactions. One person's actions are portrayed as explicitly evoking the other person's actions. These complementary transactions, in turn, are organized into self-perpetuating maladaptive interpersonal patterns that are characterized by rigidity and chronic repetitiveness (Kiesler, 1996; Schacht et al., 1984; Wachtel, 1993). Whereas past events may activate these maladaptive patterns, their cyclic nature sustains them.[5]

This narrative structure is called the cyclical maladaptive pattern (CMP; Schacht et al., 1984). It overlaps extensively with a formulation model, the Core Conflict Relationship Themes (CCRT; Luborsky & Crits-Christoph, 1997), which has undergone extensive reliability and validity studies. Luborsky and his colleagues have convincingly demonstrated that the CCRT embodies a "central relationship theme" that influences interpretation of, and conduct within, a wide range of interpersonal settings (Luborsky & Crits-Christoph, 1997). Clinicians using the CMP or the CCRT are likely to come up with very similar interpersonal themes for the same patient (Johnson, Papp, Schacht, Mellon, & Strupp, 1989). According to Levenson and Strupp (1997, p. 91), the CMP is

> a plausible narrative incorporating major components of a person's current and historical interactive world. . . . It describes the nature of the problem, leads to the delineation of the goals, serves as a guide for interventions, enables the therapist to anticipate reenactments within the context of the therapeutic interaction, and provides a way to assess whether the therapy is on the right track. . . .

Like the CCRT, the CMP includes intrapsychic components (i.e., wishes and intentions that can be incompatible with each other and can evoke expectations of negative responses from others) and inter-personal components (i.e., conflicts between one's actions and the actions, real or imagined, of others; Book, 1998; Luborsky, 1997a; Strupp & Binder, 1984). The CMP is a conceptual model representing:

> a central or salient pattern of interpersonal roles in which patients un-consciously cast themselves, the complementary roles in which they cast others, and the maladaptive interaction sequences, self-defeating expectations, and negative self-appraisals that result. (Schacht et al., 1984, p. 68)

The CMP is an application of the relational theories of personality and psychopathology described in Chapter 2. It represents a cognitive map of a circumscribed area of the patient's dysfunctional mental activities and maladaptive interpersonal behavior, which can guide the therapist's approach to the patient. This formulation model reflects a theoretical view in which dysfunctional mental activity, maladaptive interpersonal behavior, and the restricted range of reactions evoked from others interact reciprocally. Thus, a CMP depicts psychopathology as self-perpetuating, regardless of its origins. The model consists of four interrelated categories:

1. *Acts of Self:* Overt and covert (mental) acts. This category emphasizes wishes and intentions (e.g., "I want to be loved. I am planning to speak my mind.").
2. *Expectations of Others:* Assumptions, anticipations, and expectations about how others are going to respond to the person, particularly with reference to the person's acts (e.g., "Others will probably disapprove of my speaking my mind.").
3. *Perceived Acts of Others:* Recollections and reports about the actions and intentions of others. These perceptions tend to be subject to misinterpretation because of the influence of the person's expectations of others, particularly with reference to the person's acts (e.g., "She did not respond to my expressed opinion, which probably meant that she disapproved of it.").
4. *Self-Image and Self-Treatment:* The view of oneself and the ways one treats oneself, particularly with reference to one's actions and perceptions of how others have responded (e.g., "I could

kick myself for expressing my stupid opinions, because she must have thought I sounded ignorant.").

Extensive theoretical and clinical discussions of the CMP can be found in previous works (e.g., Binder & Strupp, 1991; Butler et al., 1997; Levenson, 1995; Strupp & Binder, 1984).[6] An example of the type of individualized problematic story that is generated with the CMP format is provided by information from Carl's treatment, described earlier in this chapter.

PRESENTING PROBLEMS

Carl complained that he felt uncomfortable and out of place with other people. He felt as if he had some sort of emotional barrier between himself and others, and he had no friends. This barrier was particularly distressing with his wife and small child. Carl did not spontaneously complain of any symptoms but when asked, he described a chronic despondency associated with his interpersonal problems.

> *Acts of Self*: The patient desires acceptance from others. He wishes to establish close relationships with his immediate family and to make friends. However, the patient does not let others know of his desire for closeness.
> *Expectations of Others*: The patient expects to be criticized by others for having selfish aims.
> *Perceived Acts of Others*: When other people do not explicitly convey acceptance and friendliness, the patient perceives them as feeling imposed upon by him and then ignoring and rejecting him.
> *Self-Image and Self-Treatment*: The patient believes that his needs and motives are selfish. He constricts his own emotional experience.

CONSTRUCTING A CYCLICAL MALADAPTIVE PATTERN

Transforming information about an individual's subjective distress and impaired functioning into a formulation about a circumscribed problematic situation requires a collaborative effort between therapist and patient. The therapist encourages the patient to talk about his or her distressing experiences and about life, in general. The therapist responds with questions, observations, comments, and possible explanations, and encourages the patient to revise and correct any interpretations of the meanings of events in his or her life. Guided by a theoretical framework for understanding personality and psychopathology and by the products of this reflective conversation with the patient, the therapist proposes a synopsis of the problems, sometimes including a hypothetical explanation for them. This synopsis is the initial case formulation, which in brief dynamic–interpersonal psychotherapy takes the form of a CMP.

In order to generate clinical data that are relevant to constructing a CMP, the patient must be encouraged to provide anecdotes about interactions with other persons (Book, 1998; Luborsky & Crits-Christoph, 1997). If the patient tends to focus on discrete actions, symptoms, or subjective experiences, he or she is encouraged to describe the interpersonal context in which behaviors as well as physical and psychological experiences occur. There are four prototypic questions, corresponding to the four CMP categories, that frequently can serve as guidelines for generating content to illuminate these categories:

1. *Acts of Self*: What are the patient's wishes and intentions regarding the other person? How does the patient behave toward the other person? What is the nature of the patient's sentiments about the other person?
2. *Expectations of Others*: What does the patient assume or expect are the other person's intentions and sentiments toward him or her?
3. *Perceived Acts of Others*: How does the patient perceive and interpret the actions and intentions of the other person? What are the patient's reactions?
4. *Self-Image and Self-Treatment*: How does the patient's experience of the interactions and relationship with the other influence the manner in which the patient views and treats him- or herself?

These prototypic questions direct the clinician to evidence of maladaptive interpersonal patterns. The patterns characterizing a particular individual, however, are constructed by a dialogue that is largely unique to the specific patient–therapist dyad. Generating specific interpersonal information as part of a therapeutic effort is essentially similar to the way in which one person learns about another in any social encounter. One person questions another, who begins to talk about him- or herself. The first person listens, becomes curious about certain details, and spontaneously asks further questions, which elicit more information. If the person listens with an attitude of curiosity, his or her context-inspired interjections will facilitate an informative inquiry.

The mental working model of the patient's central maladaptive interpersonal pattern needs to be as clear, detailed, and precise as possible. For example, the patient presents a general problem concerning conflict with persons in positions of authority whose judgments can influence the patient's life. In order to transform this relatively vague concern into a more precise problem formulation, a useful inquiry strategy is to ask about recent examples of transactions or relationships that exemplify the problem. The patient is encouraged to relate the interactions, the interpersonal context, his or her subjective experiences, and his or her perceptions of the others' subjective experiences in as much detail as possible. Relevant interpersonal content can be extracted not only from recollections of actual interpersonal encounters, but also from the manifest content of dreams and daydreams. Most patients do not spontaneously relate their dreams, nightmares, and daydreams. These mental productions, however, similar to deliberate artistic productions, reflect something about the patient's view of self and the world as he or she perceives it. Early memories serve a comparable function. Therefore, it is good practice, at propitious moments, to inquire about such mental contents, because they may reveal clues about the central issue that brought the patient into treatment at this time. Such propitious moments include, for example, times when the patient has offhandedly alluded to dreams or daydreams, or when inquiry into the patient's interpersonal experiences produce diminishing information about a preliminary central issue. When the therapist senses that he or she is embroiled with the patient in a problematic interpersonal scenario (i.e., one that deviates from a collaborative working relationship), a transference–countertransference enactment, relevant to a potential therapeutic focus, is likely taking place. The therapist searches through all of these sources of relationship episodes for evidence of a recurrent interpersonal pattern in the form of a CMP, which would constitute the central issue and the focus of treatment.

As the picture of a salient interpersonal pattern becomes more detailed and precise, it becomes easier to identify details that do not appear to mesh rationally or that are ambiguous or incompatible. Such breaks in clarity and consistency usually indicate the maladaptive nature of an interpersonal pattern. For example, a depressed and lonely young man in psychotherapy was describing conflict with a supervisor at work. This supervisor spent a good deal of time each week helping the young man master the routines of his position. Nevertheless, the young employee did not feel that the supervisor was really interested in him. The young man resented what he perceived as the supervisor's neglect of him, and this sentiment influenced his interactions with the supervisor, who was sometimes put off by the young man's manner. Such a maladaptive interpersonal pattern is characterized by inconsistencies and illogical elements that are usually not recognized and are rarely questioned by the person enacting it. *A maladaptive interpersonal pattern (and the corresponding dysfunctional mental working model) operates automatically. Assumptions and conclusions about one's experiences and actions associated with the pattern remain largely unquestioned.*

Pointing out the inconsistent and illogical components in a previously unquestioned pattern of thinking and behaving can elicit useful diagnostic information and, at the same time, instigate therapeutic self-questioning and self-reflection. While giving this feedback, however, the therapist must be alert to any indications that the patient might feel criticized. Ideally, the feedback kindles curiosity. For example, after the therapist pointed out inconsistencies in the patient's account of the relationship with his supervisor (e.g., the regular time the supervisor spent with him, in contrast to his perception of being neglected), the young employee might become puzzled and curious about why he was so convinced that the supervisor was disinterested. Once the patient's curiosity is aroused, the therapist can inquire about comparable experiences in other relationships. Once the clinician has a working model of a salient maladaptive interpersonal pattern, this model can be used as a prototype against which to check the goodness of fit with interpersonal patterns identified in other reported interactions and relationships. As mentioned above, a complementary strategy for assessing the degree of maladaptiveness of an interpersonal pattern is the amount of goodness of fit between a particular pattern and the clinician's hypothetical ideal of a healthy version of that particular interpersonal pattern. Evaluating the reasonableness, rationality, and logical consistency of an interpersonal pattern and evaluating its goodness of fit with what most people would consider a healthy pattern are both examples of applying *common sense* to the clinical effort.

Identifying a salient maladaptive interpersonal pattern is not like discovering the only thematic path in a metaphoric woods dense with interpersonal information. A more accurate analogy would depict signs of many paths, and the therapist would need to choose the one path that appears to offer the most productive route by which to understand the patient's current predicament. Choosing which interpersonal pattern to explore involves clinical judgment, which may be aided by the following criteria:

1. The narrative theme represented by the pattern provides a plausible and meaningful explanation of the patient's symptoms and other problems.
2. The components of the pattern recur frequently and with noticeable intensity (Luborsky & Crits-Christoph, 1997).
3. The pattern is part of what appears to be a predominant dysfunctional style that contributes to interpersonal difficulties (often including the therapeutic relationship) and leaves the patient feeling anxious, depressed, and unfulfilled (Book, 1998).
4. The interpersonal pattern represents a plausible, meaningful, and heuristically useful facet of the patient's life story.

AN EXAMPLE OF CONSTRUCTING A CYCLICAL MALADAPTIVE INTERPERSONAL PATTERN

The case of Jean illustrates the early sessions of a treatment. Potential components of CMP categories have been underlined. The numbers in parentheses correspond to the CMP categories. The pattern components for each of Jean's relationship episodes are grouped by CMP category in Table 3.1 on the next page. For each CMP category, the therapist searches for a recurring theme in the interpersonal pattern components across the six relationship episodes. The theme that is constructed for each CMP category is described on pages 90–91. The category themes depict a salient maladaptive interpersonal pattern.

Clinical Description

Jean has an administrative position in a medium-sized company. She sought psychotherapy because of escalating tension in the relationship with her husband. She complained of moodiness she thought was associated with her marital problems. She also complained of not doing well at work, particularly on projects in which she was not really interested. Her husband was an accountant in a company that had recently given him a significant promotion. Her father had recently retired after

TABLE 3.1. Interpersonal Pattern Themes Extracted from Relationship Episodes

CMP categories	Episode 1	Episode 2	Episode 3	Episode 4	Episode 5	Episode 6
1. Acts of self	To be recognized and valued as important; angry in reaction to feeling ignored.	To be interested in me and spend more time with me; does not directly complain.	For parents to spend more time with her and be interested in her.	Anger in reaction to not feeling acknowledged.	To be interested in me and care about me.	For others to be interested and supportive.
2. Expectations of others	Never to be acknowledged and valued.	None.	None.	None.	Others will not be interested in me.	Others will not be interested enough to support me.
3. Perceived acts of others	Not appreciated and valued.	Others don't consider me important enough to give me time.	They don't want to be bothered with me.	He is not interested in me and doesn't want to be bothered with me.	Expresses interest in me and supports me.	He seemed interested and helped me; he may like me.
4. Self-image and self-treatment	Self-defeating acts of self-neglect and self-criticism.	Self-defeating acts of self-neglect and self-criticism.	Interpersonal withdrawal, sadness, and loneliness; self-defeating attention getting.	Mood is deflated.	Uplifted when supported; otherwise, self-defeating acts of self-neglect.	Feels good when someone acts interested and supportive.

a very successful professional career, and her mother was also retired, after working intermittently during Jean's childhood.

Relationship Episodes Extracted from Therapy Session Conversations

Relationship Episode 1 (Referring to Her Husband)

"He has expressed frustration with my moodiness. (3) *He doesn't seem to feel that my work is as important as his.* (1) *It would be nice if he did.* Its kind of frustrating, because I work hard and I have a career like he does. He has done very well at his job so far, and I am proud of him. He is frustrated with me, (1) *but I get angry too when he ignores what I am doing.* (2) *I don't think he will ever think that my career is as important as his.* He's very good about doing his work. (4) *I tend to procrastinate and get down on myself."*

Relationship Episode 2 (Referring to Her Supervisor at Work)

"Yeah, I tend to procrastinate at work. (1) *My supervisor hardly ever comes by to see me.* He sends me e-mails asking about the status of my projects. (1) *My view of supervisors is that they should regularly come by and take time with you to find out about how your projects are going.* (3) *I guess I am just another employee to him* [her mood appears more deflated]. (4) *Sometimes I tend to put off work that has deadlines.* I end up hurting myself, and (4) *I get down on myself."*

Relationship Episode 3 (Referring to Her Parents When She Was Growing Up)

"They were both very busy with work and their friends. (1) *I would have liked to spend more time with them.* (3) *Once I tried to talk with my mother about it, but she seemed annoyed. It was like parenting was too boring for her. She never knew what was going on with me, who I was.* (1) *I often stayed in my room and listened to sad music.* (1) *Maybe I got back at her by dating guys she hated."*

Relationship Episode 4 (Referring to Her Therapist)

"(1) *I guess I can say that I was angry with you last session.* (3) *You seemed preoccupied with something.* After the session, my husband and I had a fight about whether or not I should go on for a graduate degree. (3) *I wondered if you think I am smart enough for graduate school. (4) I felt down a lot during the weekend.* I guess it's because I have a lot to do at work."

Relationship Episode 5 (Referring to Her Friend)

"With all that is going on in my life, (1) *I called my friend Lynn. (3) I almost cried because she seemed to drop everything to be there for me. (2) I thought that she would have more important things to do. (4) I told her that I am procrastinating at work. (3) She said that I was bright and that I should go to graduate school, and that I deserve to do better at work. (4) I felt better for a while.*"

Relationship Episode 6 (Referring to a Salesman)

"I was in a bookstore the other day. (1) *I was looking for some books on a particular topic and needed help finding them. (2) I didn't think any of the sales people would notice me. (3) A salesman did help me. He may have liked me,* I don't know. *We spent 20 minutes discussing what I was working on. (4) I felt that I was in a good mood when I left the store.*"

The Cyclical Maladaptive Pattern

1. *Acts of Self (Wishes/Intentions)*: She wants significant others to be interested in her, to acknowledge that they value her and are willing to spend time with her. She wants others to be caring and supportive. She is angry when others don't appear to be interested in her. Although sometimes she openly complains when she feels the other is not interested, characteristically she does not complain or make her wishes known, so others are not necessarily aware of her wishes and frustrations.
2. *Expectations of Others*: Others will not notice her or be interested in her. Others do not want to be bothered with her needs and wishes.
3. *Perceived Acts of Others*: Others are perceived as disinterested in her and as not wanting to be bothered with her. If the overtures of others are sufficiently demonstrative, others are perceived as interested and supportive.
4. *Self-Image and Self-Treatment*: In reaction to the perceived lack of

interest by others, she tends to feel deflated. She treats herself with self-defeating acts of self-neglect (e.g., procrastinating) and self-criticism. Sometimes she withdraws into a sad, lonely state. Either alternative may evoke withdrawal by others, which then confirms her expectation that others will not be interested in her. When others do appear interested, her mood improves and she views herself more positively.

The most straightforward way of obtaining information relevant to the construction of a CMP is by facilitating discussions about interpersonal transactions. The content of the dialogue provides literal understanding of relationship episodes. An indirect but more vivid (and sometimes more convincing) mode of obtaining this information is through "participant-observation," whereby the therapist is inadvertently recruited by the patient into playing a role in an interpersonal scenario unwittingly enacted within the therapeutic relationship (Hoffman, 1983; Strupp & Binder, 1984). By attending to his or her private experiences and to the tacit interpersonal messages conveyed by the immediate transactions between therapist and patient, the therapist can piece together a relevant interpersonal pattern. The validity of the pattern identified in this manner is supported by its goodness of fit with patterns identified in discussions of the patient's other relationships. Note that as a CMP is constructed, the content of the categories "Expectations of Others" and "Perceived Acts of Others" is particularly germane to potential countertransference roles (Levenson, 1995).

Clinical Illustration: A married, middle-aged woman in psychotherapy for depression and a troubled marriage complained of feeling uncertain about what she wanted out of life. A prominent theme was her desire to be taken care of, which was associated with the expectation that she would be chastised for this wish. She was in her second marriage. She was overweight, avoided exercise, was not attentive to the cleanliness of her clothes, and generally neglected her appearance. The patient reported that her husband complained about this self-neglect as well as the neglect of their home. She also reported that he complained about her unwillingness to deal with their marital problems. A discussion of similarities between the problems in her current marriage and her first marriage revealed that she characteristically responded to criticism by emotionally withdrawing and doing what she wanted.

The therapist had become exasperated with this patient, because she tended to dismiss the seriousness of her marital problems and generally acted as if she had no serious problems that required attention. The therapist experienced annoyance because he felt as if he was doing all of the work in the therapy. He realized that when he spoke to the patient, he sounded increasingly impatient. It appeared that the therapist had been recruited into a countertransference role in which he was provoked to chastise the patient in a manner similar to her current and previous husbands. For this patient, a CMP that includes the components "wish to be taken care of; expectation of being chastised for this wish; perception of being chastised by those from whom she seeks nurturance; and viewing herself as an unlovable burden" will aid the therapist in identifying the interpersonal meaning of his own negative sentiments toward the patient.

PRESENTING AN INITIAL FOCUS

The initial formulation of a maladaptive interpersonal pattern should convey the therapist's empathy with the patient's experience. As much as possible this formulation should present a picture of the patient's subjective world, as seen through his or her eyes. Mann's (1973) formulation of the therapeutic focus as a subjectively experienced "chronically endured pain" is similar. At the same time, identifying a chronic source of unhappiness in the form of a recurrently enacted interpersonal pattern provides a broader vision and clarity to the experience. It becomes possible to see a cursed fate as having a meaningful interpersonal structure that may be possible to alter. The patient is likely to feel understood, which contributes to the establishment of a therapeutic alliance and also (typically) raises his or her hopes. Below is the initial version of a CMP for a depressed man in his late 60s:

> The elderly patient feels that he has worked hard all of his life to be a good provider, father, and husband. He wants his loved ones to appreciate him and to act in a caring way toward him. At the same time, he expects that they will disappoint and ultimately abandon him. His loved ones raise his hopes by acting caring but end up disappointing him, which causes him to feel unlovable. The therapist proposes that they try to figure out how to break this pattern of dashed hopes and disappointments and help him to experience a greater sense of security and satisfaction. The therapist

suggests that removing his depressing circumstances will serve to reduce his depression.

The therapist may also be working toward a more complete version of the maladaptive pattern, which would include the patient's role in perpetuating it. Even if the therapist has a good idea of this more complete version, he or she may initially withhold it because the patient might react with confusion, self-criticism, or defensiveness if presented with it prematurely. Once formulated, however, this more complete version of a CMP can serve as a destination to be reached once the therapeutic alliance is sufficiently firm and the patient is sufficiently comfortable with examining his or her inner world. Below is the more complete version of the CMP for the depressed elderly man.

> The elderly patient feels that he has worked hard all of his life to be a good provider, father, and husband. He wants his loved ones to appreciate him and act in a caring way toward him. But he takes a very passive stance with regard to his own wants and needs. When he feels unappreciated or neglected, his reactive depression is expressed through a pouty, inconsolable despondency. He expects that if his loved ones raise his hopes for emotional support, they will eventually disappoint and abandon him. His loved ones may try to be helpful and compassionate, but his inconsolable and clingy manner causes even those who love him to recoil eventually, which he experiences as callous and unappreciative abandonment. He feels unlovable, depressed, alone, and he appears mistrustful and resentful.

MULTIPLE PATTERNS

For heuristic purposes, it is sometimes useful to talk as though a valid CMP will stand out unequivocally from the welter of interpersonal activity reported by a patient about his or her life. In fact, it is often possible to identify more than one recurrent interpersonal pattern evident across the range of a patient's past and current relationships, including the therapeutic relationship (Armstrong, 1980; Connolly et al., 1996). A situation may arise in which the most prominent maladaptive interpersonal pattern is identified in current and past relationships, while another tacit pattern is being enacted subtly within the patient–therapist relationship. If the transference–countertransference pattern is not significantly eroding the therapeutic alliance, then the salient CMP identified in other relationships should be pursued. On the other hand, if this CMP interferes with the therapeutic work, then dealing with it must be the first priority. It is first necessary, however, to detect these immediate influences, which are often exceedingly subtle, as shown in the following case example.

Jenny, an attractive, well-dressed woman in her late 20s, had a college degree in business and a corporate position. She sought psychotherapy for the first time because of chronic depression, which she experienced as hopelessness about finding romantic fulfillment. She reported restless sleep, sadness, and a readiness to cry in reaction to movies and TV shows that depicted good father–daughter relationships or romantic scenes between a man and woman. Her therapist was a woman. Jenny reported lifelong conflict with her father, whom she "hates." She also reported repeated conflicted and ultimately disappointing relationships with the men with whom she attempted to have romantic relationships. Her stated goals for therapy were to reduce the intensity of her negative feelings about her father and to improve the quality of her romantic relationships with men.

Jenny's parents had divorced when she and her sister were children. The sisters had lived with their mother but received little attention from her. Their mother had to work long hours to earn money for the family, because their father contributed no financial support. The sisters saw their father regularly but disliked these visits, because he did what he wanted and ignored their needs. Jenny reported that he was very blaming and complaining toward her and her sister. For example: "I try to spend time with you, but you are ungrateful. I do everything for you, and you do nothing for me." Jenny and her sister had begged their mother to reduce the frequency of these visits with their father, but while sympathetic, the mother had acted as if she were helpless in the situation. As a child, Jenny reported that she had felt selfish and horrible because of her dislike for her father. As a young adult, however, she had realized the extent of his deceit and manipulativeness, and she hated him for it. At the same time, she felt "guilty" for these hostile feelings. Jenny had a very close relationship with her mother, who always warned her about the untrustworthiness of men. As though to unwittingly prove the point, the mother had had a series of relationships with men who mistreated her.

The CMP developed and agreed upon as the therapeutic focus by this female patient and her female therapist consisted of the following components: Jenny had a chronic desire to be nurtured and protected, yearnings which she reacted to with feelings of selfishness and shameful neediness. Although she deeply desired an intimate relationship with a man, she was convinced that men were untrustworthy and exploitative and would inevitably hurt her. She also expected that those on whom she tried to rely for emotional support would criticize and disappoint her. When other people, particularly men, did treat her callously or exploit her, she was prone to believe that she deserved such treatment. She tended to react to such episodes with depression and self-devaluation.

Consistent with this CMP, the focus of therapy was Jenny's disappointment over her failures to achieve satisfying romantic relationships with men and to manage the feelings about her relationship with her father. The therapeutic work focused on similarities between Jenny's treatment by her father and the experiences she encountered in her romantic relationships. Her therapist encouraged her to realize how the most upsetting and harmful facets of the childhood relationship with her father were being reenacted in her contemporary relationships with men. Jenny's examination of these connections were accompanied by intense anger and sadness. Her sentiments about the man with whom she was recently involved exemplified her view of men, including her father: "I think it's just that he makes empty promises and he just talks so much stuff that is not true and, I guess, I'm just so sick of hearing it. . . . I hear that so much, you know, like most guys. There's so many guys who have told me so much stuff that either they haven't done or it's not true and, you know, my dad always made empty promises." The therapist's interpretive focus is exemplified by the following intervention: "You spent a long time in your life being hurt that way, being hurt by people telling you things, and you couldn't believe them, especially men, your dad, and so now it would make sense that men really irritate you and make you feel like you can't trust them."

Over a period of 12 therapy sessions, this treatment focus had evoked intense feelings of anger, disappointment, sadness, and yearning, as well as a conviction, shared by patient and therapist, that the central issue affecting this woman was her persistent enactment of self-defeating involvements with unreliable men, a pattern originally established by the relationship with her father. At the same time, there was no change in Jenny's proneness to becoming ensnared in these unsatisfying relationships with men. She and her therapist were baffled about why their accumulation of insights concerning her maladaptive interpersonal patterns with men and accompanying expression of strong feelings produced no discernible change in her behavior. Her therapist felt increasingly frustrated and ineffectual, and Jenny was increasingly disappointed with her therapist but reacted to this sentiment with guilt. She did not think it was fair to blame her therapist, who appeared to be so concerned and trying so hard. What neither of them detected was the subtle transference–countertransference enactment of a maladaptive interpersonal pattern that was related to the one identified as the therapeutic focus. This secondary pattern consisted of the role of a concerned but ineffectual female (i.e., parental) authority figure, unwittingly assumed by the female therapist and the role of an unprotected and disappointed victim (i.e., child), unwittingly assumed by the patient. Within this transference–countertransference scenario, insight and talk were depreciated currency; what the patient unconsciously sought was *substantive intervention* by the therapist to protect her from abusive men. In other words, patient and therapist were unwittingly reenacting that facet of the patient's childhood relationship with her mother in which she failed to get the protection she wanted from her father's mistreatment. Although this maladaptive interpersonal pattern was not nearly as noticeable as the agreed-upon CMP, it created a significant strain in the therapeutic alliance and, unresolved, made any therapeutic progress impossible.

THE DIFFICULTY OF CONSTRUCTING A CYCLICAL MALADAPTIVE PATTERN

In my clinical experience, I have found a positive correlation between a patient's level of maturity in interpersonal relating and the relative smoothness involved in the process of constructing a CMP. This is probably the case because correlates of interpersonal maturity, such as a coherent and richly detailed inner representational world, self-reflectiveness, good communication skills, and a reasonable degree of trust in others, facilitate the conveyance of the type of information that is crucial for constructing a CMP. On the other hand, correlates of interpersonal immaturity, such as an obtuse inner representational world and mistrust of others, impede the sort of collaborative inquiry necessary to construct a CMP (Strupp & Binder, 1984). Furthermore, patients with relatively lower levels of interpersonal maturity are more likely to ensnare therapists, unwittingly, in hostile transference–countertransference binds, thereby stunting the growth of an embryonic therapeutic alliance and the gathering of pertinent clinical information. When stymied in the construction of a CMP, the clinician should scan the interpersonal surroundings in which he or she is immersed for evidence of such a transference–countertransference scenario. Relevant clues may be right in front of the clinician's nose.

Difficulty in constructing a valid CMP (i.e., one that most plausibly and meaningfully depicts a patient's central concerns) can be created by time pressures, whether externally or internally imposed. The shorter the planned length of therapy, the more intense the pressure to rapidly determine a therapeutic focus. A case formulation may be developed without sufficient opportunity for a reflective conversation with the patient to determine the most valid therapeutic focus.

Once the therapist has constructed a preliminary picture of a CMP in his or her mind, how much of it is shared with the patient depends on the therapist's appraisal of the latter's ability to comprehend the issue and accept it. The therapist does not want to present a focus for collaborative therapeutic work that leaves the patient befuddled or feeling shamefully disposed. After establishing an initial therapeutic focus, the content of the therapist's interventions must be consistently relevant to the story embodied by the CMP. This task involves the third basic therapist competency: tracking the therapeutic content focus, which is the topic of the next chapter.

NOTES

1. The vast majority of psychotherapy research is conducted on treatments that would be considered as time-limited, regardless of whether the therapist has deliberately planned a time-limited approach.

2. Goldberg's (1992) survey of "seasoned" psychotherapists revealed that after practicing for several decades, they were more likely to appreciate how much their common sense contributed to their clinical skills and effectiveness.

3. In most instances, I do not advocate giving patients advice but prefer to use common sense in presenting alternative courses of action that may be healthier, thereby facilitating new choices for the patient. In cases of clear-cut self-destructiveness, such as remaining with a physically abusive spouse, suggestions of healthier courses of action would be relatively more directive.

4. I discuss this issue of the fate of transference in brief therapy in Chapter 2 and in more detail in Chapter 5.

5. From a relational perspective, these maladaptive interpersonal patterns are the overt expression of dysfunctional mental working models of the interpersonal situation.
6. For the definitive review of this work, see Luborsky and Crits-Christoph (1997).

4

Competency 3

Tracking the Issue That Is the Focus of Therapy

A therapist must attempt to work on the patient's problems consistently within the explanatory framework provided by the initial case formulation. For the dynamic–interpersonal brief therapist, this task involves explicating the contribution of a salient dysfunctional mental working model and corresponding maladaptive interpersonal pattern.[1] This interpersonal pattern and components of the underlying dysfunctional mental working model comprise the CMP (described in Chapter 3). Evidence that the therapist is diligently tracking the CMP is found in the content of his or her interventions; this content is consistently relevant to an interpersonal theme that has been designated as exerting a particularly maladaptive influence on the patient's life.

There is reasonably good research evidence that tracking a therapeutic focus in the form of a salient maladaptive interpersonal theme contributes to positive treatment outcome. Several empirical studies, representing different forms of time-limited psychodynamic therapy, have reported that a consistent correspondence between the content of therapist interventions and the interpersonal theme reflected in an identified therapeutic focus is significantly associated with positive treatment outcome, regardless of type of interventions used (Crits-Christoph, Barber, & Kurcias, 1993; Crits-Christoph et al., 1988; Norville, Sampson, & Weiss, 1996; Piper et al., 1993; Silberschatz et al., 1986).[2] Another source of evidence for the importance of tracking focal themes comes from research on the activities of expert or "master" therapists during portions of therapy sessions that they consider to be significant for conducing change. These experts consider tracking a salient interpersonal theme across relationships (i.e., horizontal interpersonal pattern recognition) and across time (i.e., vertical interpersonal pattern recognition) to be important to the therapeutic change process (Goldfried et al., 1998).

A brief therapy in which the therapist constructs a precisely structured focus will probably show relatively little change in that focus. Conversely, a longer treatment in which the focus is broader and more abstract will likely have more digressions from the initial focus (Hatcher, Huebner, & Zakin, 1986; Hoglend & Piper, 1995). Even when the therapeutic focus is on one salient, pervasive interpersonal theme, the initial depiction of this theme is likely to undergo modifications over time, as the therapist refocuses his or her mental picture (i.e., working model) of the patient based on new information and understandings (Hatcher et al., 1986; Madill & Barkham, 1997). Also, the case formulation constructed by the therapist in his or her mind may not be in the same form as the one he or she initially presents to the patient. The therapist may decide that the patient is ready to accept only a limited version of the formulation, or the therapist may have less confidence in the more speculative parts of the formulation. In sum, the available evidence indicates that treatment outcome is enhanced by a strategy of tracking a structured content focus combined with flexibly modifying the content as new information arises and digressing from the initial focus as circumstances dictate.

In brief psychotherapies the pressure to achieve something quickly may cause the therapist to try to extract progress out of a focal issue that initially seemed promising but turned out to have less-than-expected therapeutic relevance. More often, however, therapists have a difficult time sticking to a focal issue even when it proves to be highly relevant. Evidence suggests that therapists generally are not particularly skilled at the task of tracking a therapeutic focus; specifically, they reveal a surprising lack of consistency (Crits-Christoph et al., 1988, 1993). Although flexibly adjusting one's attention to changing circumstances is important, it appears that too many therapists are more than flexible. Their pictures of the relevant issues in therapy are too diffuse, and they may be prone to wander about, without clear maps to guide their journeys. Psychotherapy training programs need to cultivate the development of those skills required to track a therapeutic focus more effectively. Also, independent practitioners need to be more disciplined in striving to consistently track a focal theme in the therapies that they conduct.

STRATEGIES FOR TRACKING A THERAPEUTIC FOCUS

A key component of tracking a focus consistently is having as clear, coherent, and precisely detailed an initial formulation as possible to track. As discussed in detail in Chapter 3, in dynamic–interpersonal psychotherapy the formulation is framed as an interpersonal narrative that reflects a dysfunctional mental working model and corresponding maladaptive interpersonal pattern. In order for the therapist to construct and track such a formulation, he or she must repeatedly encourage the patient to produce interpersonal information. Regardless of the types of intervention used (e.g., questions, reflections, clarifications, interpretations), the aim of the intervention should be to generate, clarify, and elaborate interpersonally relevant information. As also discussed above, a mind-set of curiosity is a good foundation upon which to develop skills at eliciting narratives from a patient. In the broadest terms, the object of the therapist's curiosity is some interpersonal scenario with which the patient is engaged at the moment. The aim is always to bring the picture of an interpersonal scene into sharp focus as quickly as possible. The sharper the clarity and the more elaborate the detail of any particular scene, the easier it will be to analyze it and compare it to other scenes, in the search for salient repetitive patterns.

The interpersonal pattern recognition skills required for tracking a content focus have been developed and refined, to varying extent, long before a therapist begins to do psychotherapy. The perception of interpersonal plots and themes and the assignment of meaning to them are skills exercised in making sense of movies, plays, books, poems, song lyrics, and personal relationships. We practice these interpersonal pattern recognition skills ubiquitously, without realizing it, before we become therapists as well as after.

The therapist's mental working model serves as a map for tracking this interpersonal theme through the often-confusing terrain of the patient's mind. This working model is a mental picture, a conceptual template, that depicts a specific interpersonal scenario. All subsequent interpersonal scenarios associated with the patient are transformed in the therapist's mind into templates that can be superimposed on the prime template, to compare for goodness of fit. A relevant fit does not require the scenarios to be identical. It is sufficient for an examined scenario to be similar to the prototypic scenario in fundamental ingredients. Judging the similarity (or lack thereof) between two scenarios is a facet of therapeutic competence that improves with experience.

Do not underestimate the degree of mental discipline that is required to search for and identify evidence of a salient interpersonal theme throughout the patient's communications. With sufficient practice, it is not so much mental effort that is required as an easy, open receptivity. The discipline is manifested primarily in maintaining the appropriate mind-set, reflected by an ever-present question in the back of the therapist's awareness: "Where is the central issue, the thematic focus, now?" Evidence of a focal interpersonal theme can be found in the content of the patient's communications as well as embedded in tacit interpersonal messages nonverbally conveyed between patient and therapist (e.g., a therapist and patient both slouching back in their chairs may convey the message that they have agreed to emotionally disengage from their collaborative work because they both feel that it is not going anywhere). A salient interpersonal theme persists across sessions; it is like the plots of a television soap opera: you can resume watching one of these "soaps" after an extended hiatus and quickly recognize a variation of the same story line that was center stage the last time you watched. Therefore, it is useful to begin each session with the assumption that what is talked about and what transpires reflects a seamless continuation of the issues that were salient at the end of the last session. Look for the logical implications of the situation in whatever the patient is talking about, but particularly when the topic appears emotionally loaded. Often the results will lead back to the central issue of the treatment. When extrapolating the implications of a topic, rely on common sense as well as personal and professional experiences and knowledge.

Although maladaptive interpersonal patterns do tend to repeat themselves, not every element of the focal interpersonal theme is detected in every session. If the therapist maintains a sharp watch, he or she is more likely to spot enough examples of a salient theme to convince the patient of its influence. Each time the therapist identifies the presence of a salient interpersonal pattern, he or she models the skill of pattern recognition and, at least indirectly, coaches the patient in practicing the important skill of self-reflection. In time, the patient can become more skillful at self-monitoring for their particular interpersonal pattern.

Obviously people vary in their ability to identify and follow an interpersonal theme. Like having perfect pitch for music, some people are naturally gifted at following interpersonal themes, whereas others appear to be have great difficulty at it. At the extreme, some people (including some therapists) appear to be interpersonally "tone deaf." As is the case in any domain of complex performance, regardless of variations in natural ability, to achieve and maintain the highest level of proficiency at interpersonal pattern recognition and tracking requires disciplined practice (Ericsson & Charness, 1999).[3] A person who is highly proficient at this skill appears to perform it relatively effortlessly. But this external appearance of ease may hide intense, focused, mental discipline.

Sometimes when a subtle transference pattern is active, not even an experienced therapist is immediately aware of its influence on his or her interactions with the patient. The following case illustrates such a transference pattern.

Norman was a middle-aged divorced man who sought psychotherapy because he felt that his supervisors at work were unsupportive and overly critical. He feared that his attitude was evident and could jeopardize his employment. In his personal life, Norman was isolated. He had been divorced for many years, and he rarely saw his grown children and had limited social contacts. The primary issue on which the therapeutic work focused was his chronic pattern of extreme self-sufficiency. The apparent origin of this interpersonal pattern was his family. His parents had been reliable providers but had promoted an interpersonal style of avoiding personal issues and withholding any guidance about personal matters with their children (Norman, his brother, and sister). If anyone in the family showed any need for emotional support or guidance (e.g., regarding educational decisions), his father would ridicule him or her.

His therapist developed the following CMP to guide his work: Norman wished for understanding and support from significant others. He expected, however, to be mocked and rebuffed if he exposed these wishes. He tended to misinterpret the overtures of others as inevitably leading to intrusive actions and criticism, and he responded by proactive irritability and/or by emotional and interpersonal withdrawal. These responses left him feeling inept and worthless.

After several sessions of psychotherapy, Norman realized that he tended to transpose onto his work relationships the same sort of expectations he had about his family relationships: (1) He assumed that he would not be supported at work by supervisors or peers, (2) he misinterpreted their attempts to be helpful as intrusive or critical, and (3) he assumed that his supervisors would ridicule him for wanting help. These sentiments were the source of his standoffish and contentious manner at work. Once Norman began to examine the parallels between his work problems and his childhood family experiences, his work situation improved, and he expressed a desire to focus in therapy on his social isolation.

After about 10 sessions of successful work on his employment problems, Norman evidenced a mild idealized paternal transference toward his male therapist, whom he viewed as wise and supportive. He made repeated subtle efforts to obtain advice from his therapist about how to improve his social life. His therapist sought to balance attempts to draw Norman's attention to his struggles around seeking support from others, such as his therapist, with the provision of some opinions about the issues raised by him. The patient's ambivalence about seeking support and guidance from others was continually evident. He spoke with regret about letting down his children by not providing sufficient support and guidance, but he also ridiculed as "silly" his desire for support from his male therapist. Although Norman was usually quite perceptive about his own behavior, he repeatedly was surprised when his therapist pointed out the parallels between his recollections of being ridiculed as a child by family members for seeking support and his own self-ridicule about the same issue.

In a session following a particularly strong transference enactment of this issue, Norman expressed a concern that his supervisors at work thought that he "didn't have the balls" to take on more responsibility. He expressed curiosity about his therapist's opinion of his ability to take on more responsibility, but he avoided any direct question. The therapist made reassuring comments about Norman's abilities, based on the patient's descriptions of his work performance, but failed to see that the issue probably represented a variation of the major thematic focus: namely, Norman's long languishing desire for emotional support and guidance, which was associated with ridicule as a child, was now associated in Norman's mind with weakness and lack of ability.

This example illustrates not only how a therapist can identify parts of a transference enactment while missing other parts, it also illustrates how prominent interpersonal patterns, including transference enactments, are evident across sessions. As I mentioned earlier, a useful mind-set for tracking a focal interpersonal pattern is to view each session as directly unfolding from the previous session. Regardless of the amount of time between sessions, a focal interpersonal issue or pattern appears like a seamless narrative.

Tracking a therapeutic focus is facilitated by constructing the sharpest possible mental picture of the focal interpersonal pattern. In this effort, Strupp and Binder (1984) used the term "disciplined naivety" to refer to the scrupulous avoidance of assumptions about interpersonal meanings and an equally scrupulous attention to details about the patient's reported experiences. The therapist should not hesitate to ask questions, even about the slightest nuances of interpersonal events. At the same time, the therapist must sift through information, deciding what is relevant to the therapeutic focus. This is a process of "selective attention and selective neglect" (Balint et al., 1972) in what often is experienced as a welter of clinical material.

Even novice therapists can use their previous life experiences to help detect a CMP in the patient's reports of his or her interpersonal encounters. As a patient talks about a particular interaction, the therapist constructs a working model of a healthy prototype of the class of relationships to which the patient is referring; for example, a romantic attachment, a close family member, a friend, a business contact. The therapist also constructs a mental template of the particular interaction or relationship about which the patient is currently talking. Then, the therapist mentally superimposes these two mental templates over each other, in order to appraise the goodness of fit. Clues about a relevant maladaptive interpersonal pattern (i.e., CMP) are highlighted in the discrepancies between the two templates.

AN EXAMPLE OF TRACKING
A CYCLICAL MALADAPTIVE PATTERN

In Chapter 3, we encountered Carl, who felt an uncomfortable emotional barrier between himself and other people, including his wife and young child. In the first therapy session, his descriptions of an attempt to join his church's musical group and of his relationships with colleagues at work revealed the core of a maladaptive interpersonal pattern which became the initial therapeutic focus, in the form of a CMP: Carl desired acceptance from others. He wanted to establish close relationships with his immediate family and to make friends. However, he hid his desire for closeness from others. He expected other people to view him as selfish for having personal desires, particularly a desire for interpersonal closeness. When other people did not explicitly convey acceptance and approval, he assumed they would feel imposed upon by him, and he misperceived them as ignoring and rejecting him. He was prone to self-criticalness, especially regarding his own interpersonal desires. In order to protect himself from exposing what he considered to be shameful desires and feelings, he characteristically constricted his emotions and desires.

In subsequent sessions, Carl described facets of his childhood experiences that provided a hypothesized origin of his conflicts around interpersonal intimacy. His parents were good providers and successful in their respective careers. Neither of them, however, was comfortable with emotional closeness or with conveying personal feelings. Carl's father was especially uncomfortable with personal issues, although his career accomplishments and strong personality made him an imposing figure of admiration and respect to his son. At the same time, Carl's father could be very intimidating, particularly when he used biting sarcasm to express his displeasure at a family member. Carl had always longed for a closer relationship with his father. Failing to satisfy this wish, as a young man he had engaged in various rebellious acts that could be viewed as attempts to provoke his father into paying more attention to him. Carl eventually settled into a stable, successful career and stifled his desire for closeness—with anyone.

This information about Carl's father was provided during one session early in treatment, during which his father was the primary topic. Carl and his therapist subsequently did not meet for 2 weeks because the latter was out of town. What transpired in the next session illustrates how a focal interpersonal theme exerts its influence, usually connecting sessions over time in a seamless narrative. It began with Carl asking his therapist whether they should address each other with first or last names. Carl was unable to articulate why he had brought up the subject, although he admitted that the nature of his relationship with his therapist had been on his mind since the first session. He also admitted that he would prefer that they called each other by first names, because that would be "more informal and relaxed, and friendly." His therapist inquired about this implication.

T: Do you feel that last names would be formal and unfriendly?

P: (*Laughs.*) Somewhat.

T: What would be unfriendly about it?

P: Well, last names imply a more formal relationship, more distant. Not so much unfriendly as cooler or more distant.

By this time, the therapist had created a working model of the current interaction that was characterized by a negotiation around interpersonal closeness, with the patient desiring more of it. The therapist also had a mental template of the patient's relationship with his father, which was characterized by a frustrating barrier that limited closeness. Superimposing these mental templates revealed a connection to the therapist, a transference enactment in which the patient was seeking closeness to the therapist, and the therapist was being recruited into the countertransference role (see Strupp & Binder, 1984) of an aloof father. For Carl, first or last names symbolized the amount of interpersonal closeness that would be allowed. The therapist realized that by responding that he routinely used last names in this kind of professional relationship, he would be facilitating his recruitment into the role already unwittingly assigned to him in this scenario. Nevertheless, the therapist did inform Carl of his preference. He made this decision because it was consistent with his usual practice, he judged the initial therapeutic alliance to be sufficiently firm to withstand any strain that might result, and he anticipated that his action would highlight the central issue around Carl's father that was influencing the therapeutic relationship.

T: In this situation, customarily I have gone by last names.

P: OK, I just needed to know what the arrangement should be.

T: In the context of what you have been saying about the implications of names, what reaction do you have to that?

P: This may be my assumption, but you seem to have a pretty distant approach to me. You don't show much emotion, and you are pretty analytical. This is my gut reaction, but it makes sense to me. It goes along with my impression of you.

T: How do you feel about it?

P: I'm sort of uncomfortable with it, like with the whole approach. I always feel a little ill at ease and wishing that I could break through that sense of reserve that I get from you.

T: Can you elaborate on both of those experiences? You feel ill at ease, and you also want to break through what you see as my reserve.

This therapist, in fact, had a relatively "reserved" interpersonal style. It would have been more in the spirit of a collaborative, constructivistic dialogue had he "owned" his reserve directly rather than implying that it was merely the patient's view (i.e., ". . . *what you see* as my reserve"). The transferential misinterpretation is not in the perception of the reserve but rather in the idiosyncratic implications for the patient, such as that the therapist will not approve of Carl's desire for greater interpersonal closeness.

P: The ill-at-ease part is that I want to know what you're thinking. I would like to have some more direction and some more concrete *something* to hang on to. But it seems that no matter what I do to try and get it, you manage to maintain the same attitude that inspired me to want it. In other words, like I'll say, "I often wonder if you like me," and I'll say, "Well, do you like me?" And you say, "Well, why do you think this matters to you?" So I don't get what I am after . . . and then I have to keep trying or just give up. I try various things to unseat you from your attitude, but nothing works.

The therapist reflected the patient's main point and wondered about the implications.

T: If I am hearing you right, it sounds like you are increasingly sensitive to what I think of you or feel about you. And it also sounds like you are increasingly sensitive to what you feel is my *reserve*. There is something about it that is very discomforting for you, or frustrating. I'm not sure those are the right adjectives.

P: *Uncomfortable* sounds right, but there is something *discomforting* about it too. I have the idea in my mind that since my goal for coming into therapy is to learn something about how to relate to people, and in particular how to become friends with people, that maybe I am feeling that if I am not doing that with you, maybe the therapy isn't really working, or I'm not doing what I came here to do. (*Laughs anxiously.*)

This was the first instance in which Carl complained, even indirectly, about his therapist's treatment of him. In particular, the patient is implicitly complaining that he has been rebuffed by his therapist and consequently would not accomplish anything in therapy. A short time later, Carl continued his complaints about the therapist's interpersonal reserve. This point in the session clearly exemplifies a "therapeutic alliance rupture" (Safran & Muran, 2000).

P: I feel that this is a more direct personal confrontation with you, and I would expect you to possibly have more feelings about it than, say, about my family. This is something that directly concerns you. I'm talking about *you*, and about my experience with you, and how I experience the therapy. I think our relationship should have more back and forth. If I'm talking about my family, you can point things out, provide explanations. But here it seems like I'm expecting a different type of give and take because the topic is 50% you.

T: What makes you feel like we are having a confrontation?

P: I guess, to me, the fact that I am telling you that I am uncomfortable and that I have the feeling that, to an extent, I am not getting what I came here for, and that's what my discomfort is stemming from. To me it seems like a challenge to you. Like you either justify your actions or persuade me that everything is OK, or in some way respond to my dissatisfaction with my experience.

T: You mean, with me?

P: With, well, OK, with you. (*Laughs.*)

The therapist was willing to accept Carl's criticism and complaints. He did not become defensive, nor did he try to sugarcoat the immediate interpersonal strains with vague and unsubstantial reassurances. When Carl began to evidence cold feet about directly confronting the therapist—a common reaction during an alliance rupture (Safran & Muran, 2000)—the therapist encouraged him to continue explicitly airing his sentiments. Carl again admitted that he was dissatisfied with the therapist's interpersonal "reserve." Further inquiry by the therapist about Carl's reaction to his reserve led Carl to admit the following:

P: For my part, I would say that I probably am hanging back and not mentioning things as they come up. I'm letting things develop and not really letting you hook into me.

T: Why do you think you are doing that? What do you think holds you back?

P: Some kind of risk involved, and I'm not wanting to make waves, and I'm feeling like I'd rather, to an extent, adjust to what your expectations are of the situation.

T: Why? Especially since you feel that *you* are dissatisfied with *me*.

P: Well, yes, I don't know. Why would I be holding back? It's because, like I said about the names, maybe [the relationship] would develop more and I wouldn't have to say anything about it, which would be easier. I wouldn't have to bring up something that is uncomfortable, risk your displeasure or making you uncomfortable, or whatever.

In the therapist's mind, the templates characterizing his current interaction with Carl and Carl's relationship with his father have a close fit. The therapist, however, chose not to make a linking transference interpretation ("transference/parent link"; Malan, 1976a) at this point, because the reality of his interpersonal reserve and his informing Carl about his preference for last names created a high plausibility for Carl's view of their relationship as distant and formal. Carl had some valid reasons for complaining, if his goal was to practice feeling close to people. The therapist's technical strategy was to examine the idiosyncratic implications of Carl's view of their relationship. These implications carry the transferential meanings of the relationship.

T: If we pull together some of these observations and experience you have described in the last few minutes, maybe it would help us understand particularly what makes you hold back. You see me as reserved, and you see yourself as holding back because you are not sure what that reserve is about, and you feel a risk and are anxious about it. You are also very reluctant to make waves. If you were going to say you were dissatisfied, you don't want to make it personal. It's hard for you to admit that you are dissatisfied with me. Once you did, of course, you said, "It's not only you. It's 50% me." I wonder if you don't read something into my reserve that is, one, that I don't like you, and two, that I don't want to be bothered by your feelings, particularly if you've got something to complain about, fuss about—any feelings, whether they are your feelings of wanting to be closer to me or your feelings of dissatisfaction, your complaints. So you feel a need to hold back, because otherwise I would get mad and be offended, and our relationship would be ruined.

P: I think that's true.

These interchanges and the therapist's here-and-now transference interpretation capture a variation of the central issue formulated with the CMP model: the wished-for closeness, the expectation of rebuff, and the inhibition associated with a self-judgment of selfish motives. The therapist focused on Carl's defensive "holding back" because this facet of the maladaptive interpersonal pattern appeared to be the immediate source of the emotional barrier that was the incentive for Carl seeking treatment.

Over the next 2 months of weekly sessions, this focal theme was systematically examined. During this time, a character trait was identified that reinforced the defensive "holding back" that contributed to Carl's sense of an emotional barrier between himself and others. In his dealings with others, particularly his wife and child, he evidenced an obsessive–compulsive expectancy of them to behave conscientiously, seriously, and to avoid what he considered to be "frivolities." Interpersonal closeness tends to be inhibited when humor and playfulness are disparaged. Carl summarized his progress in this area early in the 16th session.

P: I felt like I've generally had an excellent week with my wife and my son. I think we are really getting somewhere here. I'm thinking about the things that we're [Carl and the therapist] talking about and, if nothing else, it makes me more aware when I start acting in certain ways. It makes me more able to realize at that moment that I am acting in that way. Like, if I start acting overly demanding or expect too much, I can say to myself, "Oh, yes, now, Dr. Kaufman told me my standards are very high." (*Laughs.*). When this happens, it helps reduce the conflicts with my wife. I've been spending more time talking with her and with my son. I feel like I'm more able to have fun and not be constantly watching over myself to make sure that everything is done the way I expect it should be. Like yesterday, we went out to a roller-skating rink. He's just learning to skate, and I had this impulse to try to teach him something. But I stopped myself, because I realized that my expectation was that he should practice and learn as much as he could about skating from this single experience. Instead, I just said, "No, I think we will just go around the rink, have fun, and enjoy ourselves."

Carl struggled with his "impulse" to turn all family get-togethers into something instructional or productive. For example, he was concerned that his wife had gained some weight recently and pressured her to exercise more. When she told him she felt pressured, he was more able to acknowledge his contribution. Nevertheless, Carl reported periods of time during which his habitual interpersonal barrier was diminished or absent.

P: I spent some really nice time together this week with my wife and son. My wife and I got some alone time together and watched movies on CDs. I was able to take more pleasure in just being with both of them. I knew that this was speaking directly to my problem that I am trying to work on.

Reminiscing about these affectionate moments did not last long, as Carl shifted the topic and the tone when he asked his therapist for advice concerning a disagreement with his wife. Carl's son was beginning a new school year, and Carl suggested to his wife that she walk him to school. Carl thought this would be good exercise for his wife, who had been complaining of being overweight and feeling lethargic. Carl had been frustrated with his wife for doing nothing about the source of her complaints. She, however, argued that the walk to school would be too long for their young son. Carl's therapist responded to the request for advice by encouraging an exploration of the implications of this conflict for Carl's relationship with his wife. This discussion continued for a large portion of the session, and the therapist began to wonder if it had any relevance for the CMP that had been guiding their work. When Carl voiced an offhand question about why he was making such a "big thing" about this disagreement with his wife, the therapist took the opportunity to engage him in attempting to understand why their discussion had taken the direction it had.

T: You said a minute ago that the argument between you and your wife about walking your son to school doesn't seem like such a big thing, and yet you spent the entire time today talking about it.

P: I realize when I describe it, it doesn't seem like a big thing. I feel like I have some psychological distance from it, and somehow I feel like I'm (pause), like I'm thinking about my role in the whole thing. I'm thinking that, "Here I am making this big moral issue out of it. Can I succeed at this task of getting Cynthia to lose weight?" I just feel like she should lose weight. It's only rational for her to lose weight; therefore she should lose weight. But this issue doesn't seem so important when I think about it now. I don't know why that is, exactly.

The therapist suggested to Carl that he was frustrated with his wife's inability to control her unhappy feelings about her physical condition. Carl acknowledged that he had not thought of that aspect of the issue. His attitude was that feelings should be stifled in service of doing what is rational and logical. At this point the therapist attempted to bring Carl back to center stage, by pointing out that his feelings had been put in the background while they had spent a large portion of time "analyzing" his wife.

T: Does anything come to mind from our last session, that, if you think about it, you would kind of like to put into the background and look at something else, like your wife?

P: Mm-hm.

T: Does anything come to mind from last session that might have been disturbing to you and motivated you to put your feelings in the background?

P: Well, the last thing I remember talking about was how I never really felt like I had gotten what I needed from my parents. I seem to have spent my life searching for this in somebody else and had never really found it with anybody else. I had come in here searching for it from you, searching for it with my wife. Some kind of unconditional love, acceptance. But I did not want to face this. I felt that wanting that kind of acceptance too much would drive people away. People would not be able to handle the fact that I wanted that. And it seems like we talked about how I felt that even a small desire for that acceptance was too much. And so I guess that maybe what you may be suggesting is that rather than think about that, I thought about these other things.

The predominant topic throughout most of the session had served the defensive purpose of moving patient and therapist off track, diverting them from the central theme. Once the therapist recognized this dynamic and suggested to the patient that he might be avoiding something, the latter quickly provided a nice synopsis of the CMP that put the therapeutic discussion back on track. *If the therapist is able to articulate a precise CMP and stay focused on it, the patient is more likely to develop and sustain a mental working model of this interpersonal pattern and automatically use it to organize his or her understanding of events.*

Carl observed how he had tended to focus on what he considered productive activities and projects for his family and himself to avoid facing his desire for emotional closeness. But he also reported spending more time simply being with his wife and child.

T: It's striking to me that you recall those things on your mind while we talked about your yearning to be accepted and to be loved and to be cared about. And you came in today reporting that you did spend more time with your wife and child. It was nice. But you really didn't go into any detail about that: what you did and how you felt about it. You said it was nice, but then you immediately turned to how frustrated and angry you are with this weak-willed woman who is your wife.

P: (*Chuckles.*)

T: And the picture of her struggling with her weight and how frustrating it is. She resolves to do it, but she doesn't, and then she complains about it. Why would you want anything from a person who's so conflicted and weak willed?

P: (*Chuckles.*) How could I want to be accepted and loved by a person like that?

T: Yes.

P: I do get baffled about how we get into these huge arguments, where I end up feeling discouraged, like I screwed up. I feel very confused about it, blind to what is really going on. But then we can spend good time together too.

T: So I guess the point I was trying to make in the context of what we have been talking about lately is that it seems like it's easier for you to talk about being frustrated and angry with a wife who disappoints you than it is to spend any time at all talking about the good feelings you have being with someone and who cares about you, being loved.

P: You know, what occurs to me is that my father doesn't really talk about his personal experiences. He is more likely to talk about a subject in the news or some intellectual subject, something like that. My mother will talk about her personal experiences, but they usually are complaints about something or somebody. It occurs to me that somehow or other, maybe I picked up that habit from them, that if you're going to talk about personal things, talk about things that irritate you, stupid things that other people do.

In this session, Carl created an emotional barrier in reaction to reporting affectionate, intimate experiences with his wife and child. He could not sustain those experiences, because he automatically judged them to be unacceptable. He subsequently retreated to a characteristic defensive stance of criticism and displeasure toward his wife. The influence of the CMP was still very much present: He had temporarily achieved longed-for intimacy but unconsciously judged it to be too risky and unacceptable; therefore, he had to retreat behind a defensive emotional–interpersonal barrier. Carl and his therapist, however, lost sight of it. Instead, they became immersed in the concrete details of one manifestation of the CMP (e.g., Carl's impatience with his wife's feelings about her weight) and missed the broader implications for Carl's proneness to retreat from emotional intimacy (e.g., his impatience with his wife overshadowed the closeness he had been feeling, thus creating an emotional barrier between them). When the therapist realized that they were diverging from the CMP, he enlisted the patient's help in relocating the therapeutic focus and discovered it hidden within the implications of the topic they had been examining.

AN ILLUSTRATION OF LOSING TRACK OF A FOCUS

Although the consistent tracking of a central therapeutic issue is considered to be a cardinal characteristic of time-limited psychotherapy, and there is empirical support for the positive influence of this effort on outcome, there has not been much attention devoted to the question of therapist efficacy in performing this crucial activity. As noted earlier, therapists appear to have great difficulty in tracking a focus consistently. This skill requires a proficiency in interpersonal pattern recognition that develops only as a consequence of repeated practice. Furthermore, therapists do not necessarily practice this skill while conducting treatment. Always keep in mind that an interpersonal theme often is most difficult to detect when it surfaces as an obvious implication in what the patient is saying.

What happens when a therapist repeatedly misses an important part of a therapeutic focus over the course of the treatment? The case of Sidney illustrates a therapist's oversight of a central therapeutic issue in the form of a CMP.

Presenting Problem

Sidney was a single man in his mid-30s who sought psychotherapy because of guilt feelings over not making a commitment to marry his long-time girlfriend and his ongoing work-related stress. He had had several previous unsuccessful therapies over the years. Sidney blamed himself for these previous failures, although he voiced what appeared to be indirect criticisms of his previous therapists. By his account, he was not really prepared for the commitment to work hard in his previous therapies. Although outward appearances indicated that Sidney had a successful career, going to work each day was agonizing for him. He viewed himself as incompetent and vulnerable to being exposed as a fraud. He experienced each of his promotions as placing more pressure on him, because he assumed that his superiors had increasingly higher expectations of him. He stated that he did not like his work and often thought of changing careers, but he felt stuck in his current employment for practical reasons. Sidney also experienced his girlfriend's wish to get engaged as expecting too much from him, because he felt she might be too dependent on him. Here, too, he felt stuck because he did not want to hurt her feelings. His chronic dysphoria and related symptoms indicated a dysthymic disorder, and his interpersonal inhibitions and sensitivity to criticism indicated characteristics of avoidant personality disorder.

Sidney had grown up in a small town. His parent were hard workers, but their incomes were modest. They were strict with Sidney and his siblings, expecting them to spend most of their free time doing chores rather than playing with their peers. As a small child, Sidney recalled feeling "humiliated" around his peers because he did not feel that his clothes were as nice as theirs. As a teenager, his intellectual and athletic talents led his family to expect major achievements from him, although his mother tended to be critical of him and his father. Throughout his educational and work careers, he tended to retreat from challenges or settle for mediocre performances. He had demonstrated more persistence in his current job and romantic relationship than he had ever shown.

Cyclical Maladaptive Pattern

Sidney wanted to prove that he was worthwhile by accomplishing things that would cause others to notice and admire him. He wanted to help others but also to prove that he was better than others. At the same time, he wanted to protect himself from having his self-perceived inadequacies exposed. He assumed that others would accept and respect him only through major accomplishments. Yet he felt that others expected more than he could deliver and would rather not have to deal with him, unless he pleased them. He perceived others as putting too much pressure on him to meet their expectations, in response to which he must grudgingly comply. When others were supportive and approving, Sidney believed they did not understand his failings and that he did not deserve their approval. He was ashamed of what he perceived to be his failings.

The components of the CMP that will be tracked over 16 sessions of Sidney's 25-session therapy involve his *grudging compliance to what he perceives are the burdensome and coercive expectations of others.* A case could be made that this component of his chronic and pervasive maladaptive interpersonal pattern also contributed to the failure of his previous therapies and played a role in the dismal outcome of this current therapy.

Early in the second session, Sidney castigated himself for being a "lousy" person because he thought he wanted to end the relationship with his girlfriend but had procrastinated about telling her for a long while. His response to the therapist's inquiry about his self-criticism contained elements of his grudging obligation to what he perceived as the expectations of others.

T: I mean, the way you feel about yourself is lousy. How lousy do you think you are?

P: Pretty lousy. I've stayed here in a job I don't like. I've stayed waiting for something to happen, like maybe she will marry someone else.

T: Would that make you less lousy?

P: I would feel less guilty if I knew she was OK and someone else was taking care of her. Then I could get on with my life, instead of seeing her but not marrying her just so she won't be alone. That's the way I think about it.

T: So you feel that you are not behaving appropriately or . . .

P: Yes.

T: . . . in that you continue seeing her to take care of her so she won't be lonely, or something like that? But yet, you feel like you don't want to marry her.

The therapist continued in this vein, reflecting what the patient had been saying in an empathic manner, without ever establishing explicitly and clearly that Sidney felt trapped in a sense of grudging obligation. In the fifth session, this theme recurred as Sidney recalled his years at college, where he had not performed up to his potential because he never really committed himself to his studies.

P: I just go through each day, every day, thinking that I can't get through another one.

T: Without being . . .

P: I just want to walk away from my work—I hate it! I should have left there and gone back to school to learn something that I really would have enjoyed. I feel like my college education was a waste, because I wasn't studying what I wanted, but I didn't really know what I would enjoy. During college, I had one run-in with a girl. She came up to me and initiated a conversation. And it's always been like that. I had a hard time meeting girls. I went to this bar with a couple of friends of mine. This girl came up to me, and we ended up having sex over several weeks. She wanted me to spend time helping her out around her apartment. But then she wasn't so available, and I was glad that it ended.

Sidney talked for a few more minutes about his undergraduate college experiences. He then described his thwarted desires to go on to graduate school. He had wanted to obtain a master's degree in business but felt obliged to give up that dream temporarily because of family responsibilities.

P: I went back home to live with my parents because my mother was sick. I knew I wanted to go back to school, that's all. I didn't want to live where my parents lived, but my mother was very sick; she was dying, and my father asked me to come live at home. So I did.

Sidney continued to relate his experiences after college of feeling trapped by family obligations for several more minutes. The therapist made no comments during this time. Sidney then began to talk about all of the things that he would have liked to do while in college and immediately after college, and about which he still daydreamed.

T: Why do you smile?

P: I have thought about this so much, it sounds ridiculous, embarrassing, but I still have it in my mind to do these things.

T: It's ridiculous. Why is it ridiculous?

P: I guess I feel that it is immature and stupid for someone my age to be talking about this. But I really think it could work. Well, I don't know.

T: I guess the thing that impressed me about it is that it very ambitious, wanting to go back to school and learn a whole new career.

During the patient's long monologue, the theme of grudging obligations first emerged implicitly in the context of his feeling trapped at a college he had not wanted to attend. Then the theme emerged implicitly around a romantic encounter, about which he was relieved when it ended. Finally, the theme emerged more explicitly in the context of family obligations that temporarily had superceded his graduate school ambitions. The therapist's eventual interventions revealed no indication that he recognized this theme of grudging obligation. His attention was directed toward what Sidney still dreamed of accomplishing.

The 16th session began with Sidney indirectly complaining about parking problems associated with getting to the therapy appointment and filling out insurance forms, then overtly complaining about his promised participation in the family activities of his girlfriend. During these opening interchanges, an implicit and subtle sense of grudging obligation can be inferred regarding Sidney's participation in the therapy. However, the therapist made no such inference. Instead, he indirectly suggested that they begin the session.

T: Well, here we are again.

P: Yeah. Not much has changed. [After 16 sessions, this appraisal is not positive and yet the patient perseveres.] It's the same old problem. Like this weekend, I had an argument with Susan [his girlfriend]. I just told her again that I was tired of the whole situation. What prompted it was a wedding for one of her relatives next weekend. I have been working a lot of weekends lately, and I'm tired of it. Now, if I don't have to work next weekend, I have to do this wedding with her. There is always something with her condo association or her family. It was a sunny day, which made me wish that I was outside doing something. Instead, she's telling me what I was going to have to do next weekend. I said I was tired of what free time I have being monopolized by her family functions. It's always something. And she said that I shouldn't go. I said that I always take her to these things, or she would be by herself. She said that I didn't have to go. But for so long I've been doing whatever she needed me to do. I guess I'll go [a blatant expression of grudging obligation!].

T: Why? She said don't go.

P: Well, she wanted me to go.

T: But then she said don't go.

P: Maybe I won't. But we have been in this rut for so long. When I have to work, I don't make any plans to do anything. But when I don't work, she's always got something for us to do, another job. Go do something with her family. I told her I was tired of working all the time at a job I didn't like. I was tired of dealing with her and her family. I am fed up with it all. I don't think I really like her family very much.

T: Do you think you don't?

The therapist focused on the inconsistency between Sidney's expressed frustration with his girlfriend and her family and his continued willingness to participate in activities with them. Eventually, the therapist suggested to Sidney that he has needs for involvement with his girlfriend of which he is not aware.

T: It puzzles me that you make it sound like all of the reasons for staying together with her are because of needs she has.

P: Yeah. That's the way it sounded.

T: And I'm assuming that there must be some needs that you have for her.

P: Uh-huh, I guess there are.

T: But that's less clear—what those needs are.

They continued to explore possible reasons why Sidney persevered in the relationship with his girlfriend. The therapist attempted to make the point that Sidney wanted the human contact but had a difficult time admitting it. His aim appeared to be to convince Sidney that he really did care about Susan. Sidney interpreted the discussion as revealing his need for human contact, in general, a need that contributed, in his view, to remaining trapped in a relationship that he really did not want. In other words, he grudgingly continued in this relationship in order to satisfy a basic human need that he could not ignore. In an interchange a short time later, the therapist still appeared to be trying to convince Sidney that he really did care about Susan more than he realized. In response, Sidney continued to express a sense of grudging obligation to work, girlfriend, and family.

P: I tell her that I hate my job. I think she hopes that that is what is making me so unhappy, and that if I could change my job, then everything would be fine. We could get married, and everything would be fine. I am afraid to change my job, because I don't know what I want to do.

T: Why do you think she has hung around with you all this time?

P: I guess we're both afraid to make contact with other people. You know, it's hard to meet new people. I've gone out of my way not to.

T: So you feel that you both have the same motivations for being with each other. But you question your motivation. Do you have questions about hers?

P: I don't think so. I think she really cares about me.

T: But you don't think you really care for her?

P: I'm afraid I don't.

T: But you're not sure?

Sidney described an incident when his girlfriend cried after he said he wouldn't be doing something with her, and he felt badly.

T: So, in a way, you care very much about how she feels.

P: I feel guilty. I feel like I'm taking care of somebody, trying to . . .

T: Well, it appears to me that maybe you need Susan a lot. How would that statement strike you?

P: Maybe I need what she gives me a lot. But I don't know if I need *her*.

T: Maybe a more accurate way of putting it is that you need her a lot, but it is very difficult to admit it to yourself. How does that strike you?

P: Well, I'm not sure. I really felt like I could get more done without her . . .

This interchange took on the tone of an argument, with Sidney unwilling to accept the idea that he wanted a relationship with his girlfriend more than he would admit. One way of interpreting the state of the therapeutic work at this point is that the therapist had become frustrated with the patient's lack of progress and was trying to impose a solution on the patient's predicament by convincing Sidney that he really did love his girlfriend. If this was the strategy, it did not work. At this relatively late stage in the treatment, the therapist continued to miss evidence of the prominent thematic component of grudging obligation to the perceived expectations of others—whether family, job, girlfriend, or therapist. The therapist's postsession comments about this exchange revealed his awareness that he was missing something in the clinical material and his growing frustration with the lack of progress with this patient. He described his struggle to find a relevant therapeutic focus and his sense that Sidney's relationship with his girlfriend might be productive to explore further. At the same time, he felt frustrated and a bit impatient with his working relationship with Sidney but decided not to explore this area with him. He also expressed pessimism about being able to help this man.

During the course of tracking a CMP, core elements of the prototype for the central maladaptive interpersonal pattern are specified and elaborated in progressively more detail as more examples of the pattern are discovered. In addition, pointing out parallel instances of this pattern's influence across relationships and across time serves to sensitize and educate the patient about the central organizing role the pattern has played in his or her life. The most therapeutically useful embodiment of the CMP to explore at any given time is located in the relationship that is the center of the patient's attention. This may be the therapeutic relationship (i.e., transference–countertransference issues), though not necessarily. In fact, in many (if not most) time-limited therapies, those areas of the patient's life that are the most emotionally arousing and meaningful to explore are current problematic relationships or past ones (Hoglend & Piper, 1995).

COMMON REASONS FOR LOSING TRACK OF THE FOCUS

The most common reason therapists lose track of the focus is that they do not remain consistently alert for signs of the central theme or issue. Their concentration drifts or their attention is caught by some immediately interesting subject or state of affairs, and they lose sight of the broader thematic implications. There are, however, several more specific types of situations that may contribute to losing track of the focus:

Patient's Interpersonal Style

The patient's interpersonal style may be vague and hard to follow. For example, Sidney had a tendency to go off on extended self-devaluing monologues that strained his therapist's concentration. For example, the themes of grudging obligations and Sidney's conviction that he would fail at everything were evident in the following interchanges that occurred in a session almost midway through the treatment. But these related themes tended to be obscured by his rambling monologues, as is the veiled implication that he also feels obligated to meet the therapist's expectations about appropriate topics to discuss.

T: Sounds like you've been going in a lot of different directions.

P: Yes. When I was in high school and then college, I would worry about exams and study and study. When I first started working, I did the same thing. When I had a job to do, I would go overboard worrying about it, especially if there was a time pressure or deadline. I thought that over the last 3 or 4 years, maybe I'd come to the realization that I didn't have to be pressured constantly. You know, that the world wasn't going to stop turning if I didn't get something done on time. But I am caught up in it again, trying to do everything. I haven't had any free time, I mean, and it's not just this job. It's been this way since Susan moved to her condominium. I worry about her being alone there. For a couple of months I didn't come around as much, and she got depressed being alone. So every day I have to talk with her about what we are going to do, and if I don't go over to her place, I have to call her several times a day to plan what we are going to do. I want to say "Can I have a night off and not feel guilty?" So much has been going on, I have trouble deciding what I should talk about.

T: I was struck by the all the responsibilities you have, your job, your girlfriend. You do a lot of looking after.

The inquiry then focused on Sidney's ambivalence about his girlfriend, and a short time later the following interchange occurred:

T: So yesterday when you were angry, you wanted to break up with her.

P: I'm afraid to admit it, because I don't want to hurt her. I feel like

I'm about ready to marry her just to get rid of the pressure. I've made myself accept stuff I don't like for years. I can do it for the rest of my life, I guess. A week ago my mind-set was that I will marry her. I decided that I could avoid my feelings about what I didn't like about her and concentrate on my job, stay busy, and it would be OK. In my new position, people sit up and listen when I say something. This is a big change for me. I am trying to get use to this and not make a big deal of it. Only a few weeks ago I felt like I didn't exist. I got to thinking that maybe the good feeling I'd been getting from dealing with these people and having been listened to—I mean, acknowledged that I existed—may be enough to feel good enough just to live, and why not just go ahead and marry her. That may be enough. I didn't have to daydream of doing something better, meeting someone better. But then when I'm by myself or when I have enough time to, like, face myself, I realize that without these other people, I would not be happy. I feel like the person you marry should make you happy, without having to have other people make you feel good. I mean, if everything else fell through, you should be satisfied with that person. That should be enough.

In the therapist's postsession records, he noted that he had felt "sleepy" during the session, as well as "disconnected" and that the patient was "fairly exhausting to grapple with."

Smokescreen Diversions

The topic of the therapeutic inquiry can become uncomfortable for the patient, who may throw up a smokescreen to avoid the content (Beutler & Harwood, 2000). This smokescreen can confuse the therapist and lead him or her off track. For example, in a session two-thirds of the way through the therapy, Sidney and his therapist were discussing his pervasive experience of failing to meet the expectations of significant others. The specific topic was Sidney's perceptions of having failed to live up to what his parents expected of him. The therapist made a relevant interpretation that even when he should feel proud of something he accomplished, Sidney tended to devalue it. This observation apparently disturbed Sidney, because he ignored it and escalated his self-devaluating comments. The therapist appeared to be thrown off course by this reaction and did not pursue his important observation about Sidney's self-devaluation.

P: My mother and father both were completely awed by anybody who had a college degree or was in a profession.

T: Would they have been in awe of their son, with a master's degree in business?

P: No.

T: Why is that?

P: They were disappointed in me, I guess. But I was the only one in my family to get a college degree.

T: And they were disappointed?

P: Yes.

T: I don't understand.

P: Maybe it was because *I* was disappointed. Well, I knew that I didn't have the confidence that I wanted to have when I graduated from college. I can remember when I left high school and thought I was going to college. I said to myself, "God, if I graduate from Central Michigan University in 4 years, I'll be confident enough to do anything I want to, so ... "

T: And by the time you got there, then ...

P: By the time I graduated, I realized that ...

T: It's kind of like you spoil anything that you touch.

P: I should have done better in school. I *could* have done better, graduated higher in my class, been a class officer.

T: Uh-huh.

P: I feel like a failure. I didn't take any pride at all in graduating.

T: Was your mother living at the time of your graduation?

Crisis Diversions

The patient may be going through a crisis that, at least temporarily, overshadows the more pervasive central issue. For example, in Laura's therapy, her central issue is her inability to assertively protect herself when being mistreated or taken advantage of by others. Then a close relative unexpectedly died, and she needed to spend a period of time in therapy grieving the loss of this important person in her life.

Breaches of the Alliance

An alliance strain or rupture causes the patient to figuratively run for cover, thus obscuring the focal theme. Most of the time, these situations involve transference–countertransference enactments that embody the central issue. Because patient and therapist are immersed in it, however, it is especially difficult for the therapist to see it. Evidence of the focal theme may be all around him or her. But often, what is right before our nose, as therapists, is sometimes the hardest to see unless we think to look for it. This state of affairs is discussed in more detail in Chapter 7.

INDIVIDUAL DIFFERENCES IN CONVEYING A CENTRAL ISSUE

The documented association between focusing on a salient content theme and positive treatment outcome obscures important individual differences. Generally, the amount and quality of clinical information produced by a patient will have an effect on the therapist's construction of a formulation. Crits-Christoph et al. (1999) found consistent differences across patients in the frequency and completeness of their interpersonal narratives in cognitive-behavioral and interpersonal therapies. Furthermore, they found that patients in interpersonal therapy, in general, produced relatively more frequent and complete narratives, which suggests, not surprisingly, that the issues emphasized by a treatment approach influence the type of material produced.

Another important individual variation concerns whether the dysfunctional interpersonal pattern that is identified as the focus of therapy noticeably influences the patient–therapist relationship in the form of transference. As noted previously, most psychodynamic brief therapies models are based on the presumption that it does (e.g., Davanaloo, 1980; Levenson, 1995; Luborsky, 1984; Malan, 1976a; Strupp & Binder, 1984). As methods have been developed to empirically investigate transference phenomena, however, evidence has emerged that partly refutes this presumption. Some patients manifest the same dysfunctional interpersonal patterns in their relationships outside of therapy as they do with their therapists. On the other hand, it appears that a majority of patients does not manifest the same salient dysfunctional interpersonal patterns in therapy that they manifest in their outside relationships and that would be considered the focus of therapy (Connolly et al., 1996). In other words, there are many patients who either do not produce useable transference material or whose transference enactments are not relevant to the focus of the treatment.

For those patients whose central therapeutic issue is found solely in relationships outside of therapy, the therapist's skill in interpersonal pattern recognition is his or her primary tool in tracking the focus. For those patients whose central therapeutic issue is also enacted as transference within the therapeutic relationship, the therapist's skills in self-reflection and self-monitoring also can be used to track the focus. In these cases, the therapist can monitor feelings evoked by the patient during sessions to help understand the transference–countertransference scenario being enacted and the role in which he or she is being unwittingly recruited by the patient (Levenson, 1995; Strupp & Binder, 1984).

Another individual difference concerns the therapeutic impact of making interventions in which the content is relevant to a salient interpersonal theme. Several studies have indicated that dealing with the content of a therapeutic focus using a consistently *interpretive* strategy has a detrimental impact on treatment outcome with patients who have relatively poor quality of interpersonal relating (as described in Chapter 3) (Hoglend & Piper, 1995). Sidney's therapy provides an illustration of this issue. Sidney viewed himself as a "fraud" whose incompetence inevitably would be exposed in his work and personal relationships. In an early session of the treatment, Sidney's therapist detected a transference implication in Sidney's extended monologue about his intense apprehension over committing himself to a position in his field: Specifically, it was very difficult for Sidney to ask for help from a therapist. The vignette begins with Sidney explaining why he remained in his job, even though he felt completely incompetent.

P: I have nothing else that I can do. If I lost this job, I wouldn't have enough confidence to go get another job. Once I quit a job with the excuse that I was going back to school. At the same time my mother passed away, and my father was ill, and his business was failing. I was working with him and going to school, supposedly. But really, I hated the job so much, I couldn't stand it. Finally, I just quit, which is not what I would normally do. That's not the way I usually behave. For a long time, I was afraid to look for another job. I didn't have enough confidence to go fill out an application for a job that required an MBA. I took a bunch of jobs that did not require much skill, no business skill. I mean, I stopped here in Omaha to see my sister on my way supposedly to another state. And I wouldn't have had the confidence to go look for a job. Her next-door neighbor offered me a job for a few weeks, and I actually earned some money. I was financially hurting by then, but I didn't tell anybody Then someone else told me about job openings in this large company. It was very hard to go down and actually fill out an application. And I didn't apply for a job in what I was really trained for. I thought it was something that I would like better, but it turned out, I didn't really like it. After about a year I got the courage to apply for a job that I was supposed to be trained to do. I got it, and my salary doubled, but I knew it would be for 6 months at most, because by then they would know that I didn't know anything. And here it is 10 years later.

T: Was it difficult to call in about seeking therapy?

P: Yes.

T: That was making an application of a sort.

P: Well, I saw your name in the phone book. Two months after seeing it, I finally called.

T: Are you saying it was a difficult call to make? Or that you move slowly, or . . .

P: I think that I have known for a long time that I should go back into therapy. My idea of the way I want to work all of this is to find some place that has everything that I want and put down roots there. And I just felt that Omaha wasn't the place. I would like to live near enough to my family to visit, but not close enough for them to know what a loser I am.

Sidney goes on quite a bit longer in this vein. As you can see, the therapist attempted to introduce a parallel between Sidney's difficulty becoming involved in a job and his difficulty applying for therapy. Sidney reacted, however, by ignoring the therapist's implications and sinking even deeper into a self-loathing monologue. Patients such as Sidney, whose capacity for interpersonal relating is poor, require extensive efforts to maintain a therapeutic alliance. Clinical material relevant to the therapeutic focus must be handled with interventions that are very clear and explicit in their meaning, as well as supportive. In this particular instance, *supportive* would mean that any parallel drawn between Sidney's apprehension about making a commitment to a job as well as to another therapy would have to clearly and explicitly acknowledge the nature of his apprehension about therapy, such as his shame at feeling like a failure again. *Supportive* would also mean explaining to Sidney that he and his therapist are working together on these problems, and that they should try to identify and discuss any impediments to working together that arise and are similar to the problems that impeded Sidney's previous therapies.

Tracking a therapeutic focus is based on the skill of interpersonal pattern recognition and, at times, the skills of self-reflection and self-monitoring. Once the therapist has identified evidence of the therapeutic focus, other skills are required to use the clinical material in a way that benefits the patient. These intervention skills are the subject of the next two chapters.

NOTES

1. The patient's mental working model is described in Chapter 2.
2. A methodological weakness in most of these studies complicates the picture, however. The ratings of therapist consistency in tracking a content focus are usually based on formulations generated post hoc by independent raters, rather than by the therapists actually conducting the treatments. The tacit epistemological assumption is that there is one content focus more accurate than any alternatives and the independent raters will discover it. This is a questionable assumption (see Garfield, 1990). A study that tested this assumption found that independent raters and treating therapists did not choose the same formulations and therefore would not necessarily track the same foci (Shefler & Tishby, 1998). If this finding is generalizable, then the meanings of the significant correlations reported are unclear in those studies that used post hoc rater-produced formulations as the gold standard for judging the content relevance of the therapists' interventions. One study, however, did find a significant positive association between the extent to which the treating therapists tracked their own focal formulations and positive outcome, at least with certain kinds of patients (Piper et al., 1993).
3. There is no research to inform us whether persons with no evident talent for following an interpersonal theme (i.e., those who are interpersonally "tone deaf") can adequately develop this crucial skill, even with extensive practice. My own impression is that they cannot. On the other hand, our training methods may be lacking.

5

Competency 4

Planning What to Do and Carrying It Out:
The Therapeutic Inquiry

A clear conception of the components of the therapeutic process, including change processes, provides a "blueprint" for constructing technical strategies that are conducive to change (Strupp & Binder, 1984). A case formulation model that is derived from a theory of personality and psychopathology provides a road map that can guide the content of technical interventions. As discussed in Chapter 1, the typical treatment manual consists of a set of "evidence-based" instructions for intervening with patients diagnosed with specific codified disorders (currently, DSM-IV-TR; American Psychiatric Association, 2000). An alternative approach, represented in this text, views proficient and effective therapeutic activity (or medical treatment) as based upon research-informed parameters but requiring, in addition, the capacity for flexibility and creativity in responding to the inevitable unanticipated exigencies of the therapeutic encounter (Beutler & Harwood, 2000; Groopman, 1999; Piper et al., 2002; Safran & Muran, 2000). Skillful therapists treat *patients*, with all of the ambiguities and complexities that characterize their lives and problems; they do not treat artificially homogenized "disorders." This view was alluded to by Strupp and Binder (1984): "In dynamic psychotherapy it is difficult, if not impossible, to make specific technical recommendations. This is true, in part, because the meaning and function of any given technical intervention are determined by the context of the therapeutic interaction" (p. 36).

Therapists choose technical interventions for a variety of reasons:

1. The therapist's theoretical orientation and training usually emphasize certain kinds of interventions over others. For example, experiential therapists favor role-playing exercises over interpretations, whereas cognitive-behavioral therapists favor assigning homework exercises over offering reflective comments.

2. The therapist's personality style creates, in part, preferences for certain techniques over others. For example, more reserved, intellectualizing therapists prefer offering traditional psychoanalytic interpretations over the self-disclosure used in experiential and interpersonal therapies by more gregarious therapists.

3. The patient's evocative style influences the type of intervention. For example, an arrogant, dismissive patient is more likely to evoke confrontational interventions or a paradoxical technique from the therapist than is a sad, poignant patient, who is more likely to evoke reflective comments and supportive advice.

4. The style of a therapist's own therapist serves as a role model or antimodel. For example, a therapist who has a personal therapist with a Socratic interviewing style may be subtly influenced to use this former's style of interacting with his or her patients. Conversely, suffering through a hostile personal therapeutic relationship may lead a therapist to make special efforts to be warm and supportive with his or her own patients.

5. Contextual circumstances dictate the use of specific techniques. For example, a sudden emotional disengagement of the patient from a therapeutic inquiry tends to evoke therapist questions about what caused this breach or, perhaps, a spontaneous decision to lengthen a session to get at the problem immediately.

The typical treatment manual dictates the techniques to be used in relatively rigid fashion. The therapist without a manual or other clear guidelines, however, may be influenced unwittingly in the choice of techniques by any combination of the above factors. A more reasonable approach, between these two extremes, is to articulate a specific strategy or plan for conducting therapy with a particular patient, while remaining open to the need to modify it as treatment unfolds. The therapeutic strategy, in turn, provides guidelines for choosing specific technical interventions—guidelines that are sufficiently flexible to accommodate improvising in response to exigencies created by the unfolding therapeutic relationship (Beutler & Harwood, 2000).

The aim of this chapter and the next is to recommend strategies that evoke and foster the therapeutic change processes (described in Chapter 2) that are the foundation of a dynamic–interpersonal model of time-limited treatment. As noted, in time-limited psychotherapy that is based on relational theory, the ultimate goal is modification of dysfunctional internal working models of interpersonal relations and corresponding maladaptive patterns of interpersonal relating. This goal is accomplished through a collaborative inquiry between therapist and patient that identifies influential interpersonal themes that organize the patient's experience and behavior. Establishing and maintaining an inquiry is the main focus of this chapter. This inquiry serves to foster the development of generic interpersonal skills that can be used to change current dysfunctional patterns of thinking and relating, as well as to fortify the patient with effective ways of dealing with future psychological strains and stresses. These generic interpersonal skills are (1) interpersonal pattern recognition, (2) self-monitoring and self-regulating, and (3) improvising in interpersonal situations. A major aim of many brief treatment models is the development or refinement of specific "coping skills" that are directly related to the patient's problems. For example, the passive patient needs to develop assertiveness skills, the dependent patient needs to develop skills in autonomous living, and the impulsive, emotionally volatile patient needs to develop self-control skills. The development of these problem-specific skills, however, is based on the use of the underlying generic skills that support the learning process. Assisting in the development of these skills is the main topic of the next chapter.

A *strategy* is a plan of action to achieve a particular goal. A therapeutic strategy serves as a guideline for deciding which techniques or interventions will be used in what way to achieve a therapeutic goal (Beutler & Harwood, 2000). The primary goal in dynamic–interpersonal time-limited psychotherapy is to facilitate the change processes postulated to occur in this form of treatment. Each change process requires a particular strategy. To recap the discussion in Chapter 2, the change processes are:

1. Cognitive insight.
2. Practice in detecting maladaptive mental and interpersonal patterns.

3. Creating new and more satisfying interpersonal experiences.
4. Internalization of new and more satisfying interpersonal experiences and the consequent modification of interpersonal schemas and corresponding internal working models of interpersonal relations.

In a typical successful therapy, change processes occur initially in a sequence from 1 through 4 and then recycle in sequences determined by the unique unfolding of the particular patient–therapist dyad. A technical intervention can serve different functions depending on the strategy it was chosen to help implement. For example, a question about a particular interpersonal interaction may serve the purpose of gaining insight into the influence of a maladaptive interaction pattern, whereas in another context the same or similar question may serve the purpose of exploring a healthier alternative form of behavior to promote a new and more constructive interpersonal experience.

Patients respond to technical strategies and specific interventions in a multitude of ways. The characteristic manner in which a patient responds to a therapist's actions is determined, in part, by the therapist's style of relating and, perhaps even more so, by the patient's personality characteristics. Psychotherapy research investigating the relationship between patient personality characteristics and treatment process and outcome has indicated that certain personality factors or dimensions influence the effectiveness of various therapeutic strategies (Beutler & Harwood, 2000; Piper et al., 2002). For example, Piper and his colleagues have convincingly demonstrated that a patient's enduring quality of interpersonal relating is predictive of his or her differential response to two broad technical strategies. Patients with relatively lower levels of interpersonal relating (see Chapter 2) respond better to a more "supportive" approach (e.g., empathic reflection, guidance, affirmation) that nurtures the therapeutic alliance (which tends to be fragile with these patients). Conversely, patients with relatively higher levels of interpersonal relating are better able to utilize a more "expressive" approach (e.g., interpretive, confrontational, affectively arousing) that is based on a preestablished solid therapeutic alliance. Luborsky (1984) explicitly emphasized these alternative technical strategies in his treatment manual describing "supportive–expressive" psychodynamic therapy.

After an extensive literature review and cross-validating research, Beutler and his colleagues developed a detailed set of guidelines for tailoring therapeutic strategies in a way that would be most effective with particular combinations of patient traits and "state" conditions (Beutler & Harwood, 2000). Beutler's guidelines tacitly emphasize the supportive–expressive strategic dimension and dissect it into several more specific strategies:

1. *Coping style.* Externalizing patients respond better to a strategy of coping skill building and symptom removal, whereas internalizing patients respond better to a strategy of promoting awareness of, and insight into, the nature and origin of psychological problems.
2. *Level of resistance.* Patients who tend to be highly resistant to the therapist's efforts to influence them respond better to a more nondirective approach, whereas patients who tend to be receptive to the therapist's influence respond better to a more directive, authoritative approach.
3. *Level of distress.* Patients who evidence a relatively high level of distress respond better to a more supportive approach, whereas patients who evidence a relatively low level of distress respond better to a more emotionally confrontational approach.

I recommend that the change process that is being fostered at the moment determine the primary technical strategy. This strategy, in turn, can be refined to match the patient's characteristics (either trait or state; see Beutler & Harwood, 2000) that appear to be contributing to his or her receptivity to influence. For example, when the aim is to promote cognitive insight in a patient who has relatively good psychological mindedness and tends to internalize problems, the technical strategy would be to foster a self-reflective inquiry into his or her mental processes and patterns of interpersonal relating. Conversely, when the aim is to promote cognitive insight in a patient who has relatively little psychological mindedness and tends to externalize the source of problems, the technical strategy might be to use a psychoeducationally toned approach to deal with a concrete situation that the patient has acknowledged as a problem. Regardless of the specific technical strategy employed at the moment, the therapist must remain mindful of the state of the therapeutic alliance and use supportive and interpretive interventions in a blend that has the best chance, in the therapist's judgment, of maintaining a solid alliance. This issue is discussed in more depth in Chapter 7.

FACILITATING COGNITIVE INSIGHT:
CONSTRUCTING A NARRATIVE THEME

We first encountered Norman, a middle-aged businessman, in Chapter 4. He initially sought psychotherapy because of his suspicious and hostile attitude toward his supervisors, which he feared would endanger his position. The central issue that was the focus of Norman's therapy was his fear that expressing a desire for emotional closeness with others would result in ridicule and rebuffs. After several sessions, the frequency of conflicts at work had diminished, and the focus of treatment shifted to his longstanding social isolation.

Several sessions into the treatment, the topic turned toward a woman whom Norman was interested in dating. One of Norman's few social outlets was a book club, to which they both belonged. Norman had talked to this woman during the club's coffee breaks, he quickly developed high hopes for the relationship—which made him very nervous: "I need to slow down and not try to get there too quickly." He described his tendency to go for long periods of time without dating and then become absorbed with one woman, rather than taking the opportunity to meet a variety of people.

At this point, we will examine the inquiry in this session. The interchanges are numbered so that my comments about them can be followed easily.

T1: From the time you've spent with her so far, what is Evelyn like as a person?

P1: I find her very interesting, and we have our love of books in common. We have talked several times about books that we both have enjoyed. I have seen her in the book club for over a year, but only recently have I found her interesting. I felt I was probably guarding myself against any thoughts or feelings that anyone else in the club would have about my dating someone from the club. I mean, that's just part of my makeup. I don't know where I get that from—I mean, if I was a completely free person and did not care about what other people thought of me, dating her wouldn't have been a consideration. But I have concerns in that regard, how I'm perceived by other people.

T2: Yes, you mentioned that before, that you had felt that somehow they would disapprove of you wanting to date somebody . . .

P2: I don't know how I imagine this, but other members of the book club would be somewhat cynical or maybe even somewhat poking fun of me if they knew. I don't know where those feelings come from, but those are the feelings that I had, and that's why I justified not calling her up and not asking her out on a date, and not inviting her out to dinner for a long time. I didn't want my feelings to be public knowledge.

T3: Poking fun of you?

P3: Well, yes. The thought that I had was, "There's Norman, and he's asking out Evelyn." I didn't think that should be anybody's business. But the way I justified it as a thought was, "Well, OK, the other people might be somewhat, judgmental." Or maybe they would be jokingly disapproving, or something like that. Like, this is a serious book club, not a dating group.

T4: So your desire to form an attachment would be disapproved of, or laughed at.

P4: Yes, right. That's exactly it. That's how I felt about it, and that's why I didn't do anything for a long time.

T5: Are you feeling that now about dating her?

P5: Well, I thought that if we did begin dating, and the book club had a social hour, and we showed up arm in arm, well, I think I would be very uncomfortable. I know that kind of thinking just messes up my thoughts, though.

T6: It seems like if you imagined this kind of a get-together at the book club, you could imagine a variety of different reactions if you and Evelyn arrived as a couple: There could be jealousy, admiration, romantic, intrigue—you know, a variety of reactions. Why do you think the only alternative that has any compelling influence on you is the idea that they would be disapproving or mocking? Two people who have known each other for an extended period of time and have a common interest find that they are attracted to each other and establish a relationship. And the only reaction you think these other people are going to have is disapproval or laughing at you. Why is that?

P6: I don't know where I get these ideas, but if I wasn't burdened with them, I would say that they would be pleased. They would be happy that two people they know shared a common interest and formed a relationship and became a couple. You know, that is a great way to look at it.

T7:   Does that kind of situation ring any bells—you know, of people being disapproving or mocking in reaction to a desire for closeness and affectionate feelings?

P7:   Well, I mean, the closest I can get to that, I guess, would be the ridicule that we have discussed in the past—the ridicule I got for expressing any feelings or emotion in my family. I guess that's where it comes from.

T8:   Yes, that occurred to me. We had talked about that before, and you had described these kinds of situations pretty vividly. Like the time your pet bird died and you were sad and cried, and your father made fun of you. That was a recurrent experience in your family: There was this kind of intolerance or ridicule of any show of feelings. And it was striking that you didn't seem to remember that immediately.

P8:   Yes, we have talked about the way my family was, so I was trying to think of other reasons.

T9:   You think it's only good for one shot?

P9:   Well, if my family experiences were the main reason, then I have to understand that is where it comes from.

T10: Although, it does sound like your recent experiences with your father have been more satisfying.

P10: Yes.

T11: But if I've heard you right, the kind of atmosphere around showing vulnerability and feelings and a desire to be close and have contact was the kind of attitude that was there in your family when you were a kid. It was a pretty harsh attitude. Your father would make fun of anyone in the family who showed gentle feelings. In that kind of atmosphere, you learn to be real wary of showing not only any feeling but any kind of need, especially to be close to another person.

P11: Yes. That's a real good word, *need*. It's a human need to be close to other people. Yeah. Well, that goes a long way to explain those feelings that I have described about my sensitivities to the way people would perceive me. It's like, you know, if they are seeing me as expressing a need or expressing a want or expressing a feeling, and that feeling is about caring about another person that you want to be with, it's kind of like that's what I would have been doing. You know, I've always been very private with those feelings.

T12: You know, well, this is kind of a speculation, but I'll share it with you and see what your reaction is. You have been really down on yourself, at least in our discussions, looking back at how you were as a husband and father, in terms of being really engrossed in your work and then partying after work. You know, really critical and regretful of letting your family down, your wife and your children. From the perspective that we're talking about now, of learning to be so very wary about feelings and needs, I wonder if one of the reasons that you did some of the things that you did while you were married and while your kids were growing up was out of a fear of feeling too close to them and allowing yourself and them to know and see any closeness and involvement? That you had to put limits on it for the reasons that we're talking about. That without necessarily being aware of it, you may have been operating from the assumption that if you really made them important to you, your wife and children, that somehow you would be rebuffed or criticized, or somehow it would end up very hurtful to you.

P12: I've never even looked at it or thought about it from that viewpoint. At this point, I can't really confirm it or say "no way." I just don't know. I just never really considered that.

T13: Well, correct me again if this doesn't resonate, but throwing yourself into your work certainly could put limits, severe limits, on how much you would feel involved with your wife and children.

P13: Yes. As I recall, my job was everything to me. It was far more important and had to come first. I put the company and their values and what they wanted and how they wanted their customers treated and serviced above my own family. My own family got what I had left, because I gave a lot of energy to the company, because I wanted to succeed. I wanted to be a good employee. The more I did the better I became, the more involved, because I was doing a good job, and I could take on more responsibilities.

T14: How much was the recognition from your superiors important to you?

P14: It was very important to me. It was very important to me that I do well, that I receive good reviews from my supervisors. And the harder I worked and the more recognition I received, the more I partied after work, before going home. You can't do that and be there for your wife and children at the same time.

T15: You described it again, from the perspective that we've been talking about today. You described a kind of a pattern of seeking approval and recognition, and acceptance and being cared about and valued at work. And by the time you get home, you're exhausted and have nothing left for your family. So that creates another barrier. You sought very little of your desire for acceptance and love and being valued from your wife and children, your most intimate relationships. So it's . . .

P15: You're saying that I didn't seek it from them?

T16: Yes, and again from the perspective that we're talking about today, one way of explaining that is that you were operating under the conviction that if you seek love and acceptance from the people who are closest to you, you're bound to be rebuffed, you're not going to get it. At best, you're going to be rebuffed. At worst, you're going to be criticized and laughed at. It's just not going to be tolerated, based on your experiences with your childhood family, and yet you seek it. So you seek it in a relatively safer environment: work.

P16: Yes, you're right. That's exactly right. I have known people who get absorbed in work, or other things, and neglect their families.

T17: Unfortunately, it is not that rare.

P17: I was absorbed in work and partying.

T18: Yes.

P18: Right. As an adult, but I'm going back to my childhood. What did I do with it then? What did I do with those feelings then? Well, if they were stymied, what did I do with them? I didn't have them, I guess.

T19: Well, you're human, so you had them. Maybe you squelched them.

P19: Yes.

T20: One important implication of what we are talking about is that what you did as a husband and father was not a reflection of an evil man but a reflection of the dilemma you thought you were in, based on your experience growing up. Namely, you want to be close, you want acceptance and approval, you want to be loved, you want to be valued, but you can't find that in your close relationships—at least, that's what you assumed, perhaps, so you have to find it in more distant work relationships.

P20: Yeah. That's very profound and very true. I can see that.

This segment illustrates components of the primary strategy implemented to facilitate cognitive insight in a patient who evidenced a relatively good capacity for interpersonal relating and introspection. The patient's inquiry into his or her life must be encouraged consistently. This inquiry is focused on elaborating the central issue, the narrative theme, associated with a prepotent dysfunctional working model of interpersonal relations and its corresponding maladaptive interpersonal pattern. Tracking an interpersonal focus (as discussed in Chapter 4) and progressively elaborating the relevant issues or themes through the examination of "relationship episodes" (Book, 1998; Luborsky & Crits-Christoph, 1997) enrich and refine the patient's focal problematic story. These focal issues must be developed into vivid, precisely detailed mental pictures in the minds of both therapist and patient. For example, Norman wished for understanding and expected rebuff. This issue appeared to inhibit his attempts to get to know his fellow book club member, Evelyn, therefore, his interactions with her were relevant to the therapeutic focus. In T1 the therapist attempts to facilitate an inquiry into a person who is central to the focal theme. In the segments T7–T11 the therapist broadens and elaborates the inquiry by linking the picture of Norman's current fears about approaching Evelyn to his recollections of his father's mocking reactions to any expressions of emotional vulnerability. The therapist acknowledged his understanding of Norman's apprehension about reaching out to Evelyn, considering what such actions evoked in some members of his family.

During the elaboration of a central narrative theme, the patient is more likely to collaborate in the process and accept the results if the therapist first attempts to develop the story as seen through the patient's eyes; in other words, to help the patient clarify and elaborate a first-person account of the life story that has absorbed him or her. The therapist can then encourage the patient to consider modified versions of the story that are not as likely to evoke guilt, shame, anxiety, and other affects that the patient is motivated to avoid. For example, in the segment of therapy with Norman depicted above, the therapist's interventions between T12 and T20 aim to help the patient see the pervasive lifelong influence of his attempts to avoid the excruciatingly painful hurt produced by reaching out to loved ones and being rebuffed. The therapist also offers a revised version of motivations influencing the patient's past behavior with his ex-wife and children: He was not a malevolent, evil man ignoring his loved ones but, rather, a conflicted man who yearned to have loving relationships but feared inevitable rebuff.

Norman's therapist attempted to facilitate a productive therapeutic inquiry through the use of both declarative and interrogative statements. From the standpoint of therapeutic impact, the traditional psychoanalytic distinctions (Greenson, 1967) among clarifications, confrontations, interpretations, and questions are artificial. Furthermore, the traditional psychoanalytic rules (Greenson, 1967) for the relative frequency of use and the sequencing of these different categories of interventions dictate an unnecessary micromanaging of the therapist's actions. All interventions should function to stimulate thinking and dialogue, to identify problematic patterns, and to practice interpersonal pattern recognition and self-monitoring—in other words, to further the therapeutic inquiry (Levenson, 1988). Clarifications, confrontations, and interpretations serve to expand a patient's awareness of internal and external experiences, each in a somewhat different way. Questions essentially serve the same purpose, often more effectively than any other type of intervention. What particular intervention is used at any given point depends on a combination of factors: (1) the patient's general style of interacting and momentary mode of coping with the immediate issue, (2) the therapist's style of promoting a therapeutic inquiry, and (3) the immediate characteristics of the patient–therapist interaction. In other words, the therapist makes rapid and sometimes spontaneous and intuitive choices about how to intervene based on what he or she thinks will be the most effective method for moving the inquiry to the next level.

In brief dynamic–interpersonal psychotherapy the heart of the problem is conceptualized as a dysfunctional mental working model and corresponding maladaptive interpersonal pattern that is hidden in plain sight. The origins of this working model and interpersonal pattern may be productively investigated only if it helps to makes sense of why the patient is thinking and acting as he or she does *now*. Always the central question is, to paraphrase the eloquent interpersonal theorist Edgar Levenson (1972), "What is going on around here?" Immersed in a repetitive maladaptive interpersonal pattern—an interpersonal rut— the patient cannot understand why life in relation to the problematic issue appears to offer so few choices. He or she cannot see the pattern, the narrative plotline, because he or she is surrounded by circumstances and characters who are, to some extent, unwittingly recruited and directed by the patient to play specific parts in what appears to be a fateful drama. Wachtel's (1993) concept of "cyclical psychodynamics" captures the inextricably intertwined actions and reactions between a person and his or her interpersonal environment that perpetuate dysfunction and unhappiness. The patient cannot figure out the immediate source of his or her unhappiness because it is all around him or her.

A good therapeutic inquiry in psychodynamic therapies often is equated with uncovering "deep" meanings, that is, arcane mental constructions that must have originated early in the life of the patient and that have become complex through a progression of developmental accretions. Undoubtedly, there are times when early experiences, as recalled by the patient, are useful to explore directly. Most of the time, however, the recollection of early experiences or the identification of interpersonal schemas and patterns that derive from them are useful as hypothetical explanations comprising part of the analysis of current problematic issues.

Wachtel (2003) has cogently argued that psychoanalytic theorizing often confounds a metaphor with the way people actually think and behave when it equates "deep" unconscious mental content with chronological origin, degree of influence, and difficulty of accessibility to awareness. He argues that a person's current psychopathology is not the direct manifestation of fixation at, or regression to, earlier developmental stages, or of developmental deficits lingering from the distant past. Regardless of how psychopathological behavior originated, it *persists* because the person continuously perceives and interacts with his or her interpersonal environment in a way that reinforces dysfunctional thinking and maladaptive modes of interacting (this self-perpetuating dynamic is represented by the CMP). Viewing the persistence of psychopathology as the result of a continuous, reciprocal, dynamic process between the person and his or her social environment has implications for time-limited psychotherapies. There is no reason to assume that psychological problems that began in early childhood must inevitably take a long time to resolve because they are deeply buried in the unconscious and, hence, will be uncovered very slowly; or because these problems must have produced profound developmental deficits that will take a long time to repair. If a patient and therapist can work together productively, they may be able to break even longstanding, ingrained maladaptive patterns in a relatively short period of time, because changing the way the patient relates to those around him or her can change the reactions evoked in others relatively quickly.

Immersion in a maladaptive interpersonal rut is supported by unquestioned assumptions and expectations, the view that things, as perceived and construed, are simply the way things have to be. Often, the reenactment of a maladaptive interpersonal pattern is so blatant that, once pointed out, the patient is astonished that he or she did not realize it. For example, a middle-aged man, Howard, sought psychotherapy for help with emotionally extracting himself from a chronic enmeshment with his ex-wife. The immediate precipitant for seeking therapy was the development of a romantic relationship that appeared to be leading toward marriage. This woman expressed concerns, however, about the extent to which Howard was absorbed in the problems created by his ex-wife. They had divorced years before, and Howard had subsequently devoted most of his emotional and financial resources to supporting his children, who had continued to live with his ex-wife. This woman was portrayed as emotionally volatile, manipulative, and hostile–dependent. Over the years she appeared to use their children to obtain extensive emotional and financial support from Howard. He appeared to be a sensitive, reflective man who was prone to assume a caretaking role with people in both personal and work-related relationships. In turn, his relationship with the male therapist had elements of a dependent role; perhaps he was looking for the fatherly guidance that was absent in his relationship with his own passive father.

The treatment helped Howard create a healthier balance between providing support for his children, who were still living with his ex-wife, and making room in his life for his current fiancée and her pre-teenage child. When Howard remarried, his ex-wife briefly escalated her hostile attempts to embroil him in her tumultuous personal life, but Howard successfully resisted these manipulations and treatment ended by mutual agreement. Approximately 1 year after the termination of therapy, Howard made an appointment to see his therapist for a "checkup." Since his remarriage, his new stepchild had become increasingly obnoxious toward Howard. With clear disgust he described how the child repeatedly manipulated his mother for attention, attempted to drive a wedge between Howard and his new wife, threw tantrums, and generally sulked. Howard was ashamed about how angry and disgusted he felt toward this child; characteristically, Howard was a compassionate and empathic person. He was astonished when his therapist pointed out the parallel between the descriptions of his new stepchild's behavior and his repeated descriptions of his ex-wife's characteristic behavior. Once this parallel was recognized, it appeared obvious to him. But he had been so immersed in reenacting the pattern of angry disgust in reaction to a desperate, hostile, manipulative other person, he had failed to recognize the familiar terrain. Howard subsequently reported a rapid improvement in his ability to respond in a calmer and more empathic (and parental) manner to his upset stepchild.

The heart of a good therapeutic inquiry—what is necessary to move it along—usually consists of sound commonsense observations, comments, and questions that point to what is going on, unnoticed, around the patient. The most obvious unquestioned assumptions and expectations about interpersonal events are often essential components of dysfunctional working interpersonal models, and yet often they are the hardest to see. For example, in the vignette from Norman's therapy (see p. 136), the therapist pointed out (at T6) how Norman, without considering other reasonable alternatives, had jumped to conclusions about how his fellow book club members would react if he took Evelyn to a club party. Norman was immediately impressed by the irrational nature of his assumptions, whereas only moments before he was convinced that his expectations were totally valid.

Norman's moment of suddenly recognizing the illogic of his thinking is characteristic of patients exploring dysfunctional working models. It is important to reiterate that, as illustrated in these clinical examples, the therapist's contribution to a productive therapeutic inquiry is often based on precisely picturing the interpersonal scene depicted by the patient and then looking for signs of inconsistency and lack of logical coherence. By making (usually silent) comparisons with his or her own personal and professional experiences, the therapist detects aspects of interpersonal patterns that do not make sense. We should never underestimate the extent to which the therapist's commonsense contributes to maintaining a productive therapeutic inquiry. To quote Edgar Levenson again, "What distinguishes the virtuoso performer from the beginner, in this field, is not metapsychological sophistication—which is often no more than locker room expertise—but the ability to make the patient move, work" (1988, p. 14).

The working model of interpersonal transactions that a patient uses to anticipate an encounter has a certain structure. This structure is represented by the CMP model that was presented in Chapter 3. The CMP provides a framework for initially depicting the central issue that will be the focus of therapy as well as for guiding the therapist's ongoing interventions. Of course, the therapist's first priority is to remain attuned and responsive to immediate contextual circumstances. Interventions are typically based on what is being discussed and occurring *at the moment*. At the same time, however, the therapist can keep in mind several generic questions that facilitate the construction of a salient maladaptive interpersonal pattern, especially during the thematic construction phases of the therapeutic inquiry. These questions can guide the content of any form of intervention and are especially useful when conducting a reconnaissance of an area of the patient's interpersonal life.

1. *What are the patient's primary intentions and wishes toward significant others?* For example, in the clinical vignette concerning Norman (p. 136), the therapist makes explicit Norman's desire for closeness, "an attachment," at T4.

2. *What are the patient's expectations concerning others' reactions to his or her wishes and intentions?* For example, at T2, T4, and T6 the therapist points out Norman's expectation that his desire for closeness, or any such overture, would be disapproved or and laughed at.

3. *How does the patient perceive the actions and intentions of others?* There were no clear examples of this sort of intervention in the vignette about Norman. The important point to keep in mind is that a dysfunctional model of interpersonal transactions is characterized by misperceptions and misinterpretations of the behavior, and especially of the intentions, of others. These misinterpretations reflect the prepotent expectations about others' reactions.

4. *How do the patient's actions, based on his or her expectations and misinterpretations of others, tend to evoke in others behavior that reinforces the patient's negative expectations?* For example, in the early phase of Norman's therapy, his therapist pointed out how his irritability toward his coworkers tended to evoke reciprocal hostility, which in turn confirmed his expectation that they would be critical of him.

5. *How does the patient's expectations and perceptions of others influence how he or she views and treats him- or herself?* For example, at T12 the therapist begins to make a connection between (1) Norman's expectation that others would rebuff his overtures for closeness, (2) his

defensive retreat from closeness with others, including his own family, and (3) his self-critical appraisal of his performance as a husband and father.

A segment from a later session of Norman's therapy provides another illustration of the usefulness of developing a precisely detailed picture of the dysfunctional internal working models of interpersonal relationships that serve to direct the patient's maladaptive behavior. As stated above, such a clear picture makes it easier for the therapist to use his or her commonsense to detect discrepancies between the patient's construal of a situation and the therapist's view of what would be reasonable or logical in the described circumstances. In this segment Norman discussed his plans for his first date with Evelyn, the woman from the book club. He was very nervous and reacted by meticulously planning the evening in his mind. He was afraid that if the evening did not go perfectly, she would lose interest in him. His concern was fueled by the fact that whereas Evelyn had an active social life, Norman had dated only sporadically for several years.

T1:   It sounds like you were dealing with your concern about not being interesting to her, until you caught yourself, by wanting to plan out the whole evening in detail—being the entertainment director.

P1:   Yes.

T2:   As you were thinking along those lines, how did you experience her? What was your view of her? What was her role in this envisioned scenario, this evening being planned.

P2:   Well, I was thinking that we could go to a movie and then get something to eat.

T3:   I don't mean so much the content of what you were thinking. You're the one who has to plan it all, this scenario. What is she doing?

P3:   When I thought about it, I realized that I don't have to plan everything. I could ask what movie she would like to see and where would she like to eat.

T4:   That sounds reasonable, but before you caught yourself and got into that frame of mind, when you were planning everything, wondering, "What movie should we see? Where should we eat?" In that frame of mind, what was her role?

P4:   I don't know how to answer that. I mean, in the back of my mind
      I was trying to be organized. You know, this is our first date. I
      have some thoughts about a movie and about a restaurant.

T5:   What if she doesn't agree with all of these plans?

P5:   We could go to a movie near where she lives.

T6:   No, I mean, you're planning this whole evening. What if you say
      "OK, let's go to this movie," and she says "No, I don't want to see
      that movie"?

Norman responded with a bunch of alternatives, indicating that
he had anticipated this possibility and had given it a great deal of
thought.

T7:   You're in this more flexible frame of mind now, but the question I
      was pursuing was to check on what appeared to be an implica-
      tion of your planning, which is that Evelyn's role is just to judge
      you. You're planning it all. It's all your responsibility. You've got
      to entertain her. Her job is just to rate you. You've got to try and
      keep her interested, otherwise she's going to find you boring, and
      she's not going to like you.

P7:   That's exactly how I felt—that she's going to be judge and jury on
      how I conduct myself during the evening and what I say and
      what I do and what we do. She's going to form opinions about all
      that, and those opinions are going to be either positive or nega-
      tive. I would like them not to be in the negative column!

T8:   So what resonates as you anticipate this date? Does what you
      have just described have any kind of familiar ring to you? Where
      does it come from?

P8:   I know I feel like I don't want to disappoint her, I don't want her
      to see me negatively. I would like her to find me interesting and
      want to see me again.

T9:   You know what occurs to me? It just struck me as you were talk-
      ing: the kind of situation that you described, that we put together,
      when we looked at it what was associated with your being seen
      at work as sort of hostile and aloof. You appear most like that
      when you feel that you have responsibility for some project or job
      and that no one will support you. You feel that they are just look-
      ing over your shoulder, waiting for you to make a mistake.

P9:   Right, yeah.

T10: They are critical of you, judging you . . .

P10: . . . collectively, all of them, because, you know, I was the one who was supposed to deal with the issue.

T11: Sounds like there's some similarity here: You assume all the responsibility for making sure that things go right, and you assume that everybody else is just standing around judging you.

In T2–T4, the therapist encourages Norman to explicate his assumptions about Evelyn's role during their anticipated date. This segment is an example of facilitating the articulation of a prepotent, dysfunctional working model of interpersonal relations. In T7 the therapist interprets the implications of Evelyn's perceived role in the working model, as constructed from Norman's assumptions and expectations. Norman, in turn, is astonished by their familiar illogic, but only after the therapist has helped him to "stand back" from them. In T9–T11 the therapist points out a parallel between the dysfunctional working model that is currently influencing Norman's thinking about his anticipated date with Evelyn and his previous construal of his work environment, which led to conflict with his coworkers and originally motivated him to seek treatment.

FACILITATING COGNITIVE INSIGHT: DECONSTRUCTING THE NARRATIVE THEME

In all forms of time-limited dynamic psychotherapy, the repeated detection and spotlighting of the thematic focus is emphasized via interpretation of the associated conflicts or issues. There is a crucial working assumption in the exploration of a focal maladaptive interpersonal pattern. Life stories that reflect basically healthy adaptations tend to be characterized by unconflicted and integrated content and coherent themes. In contrast, life stories influenced by dysfunctional internal working models tend to be characterized by (1) significant inconsistencies and contradictions in plot lines and content integration, (2) breakdowns in logical coherence, and (3) signs of conflict (Hardy et al., 1999). In a word, the stories constructed during focused therapeutic inquiries inevitably have major breakdowns in logic. They do not hold up to scrutiny guided by simple commonsense. Therefore, in the process of facilitating a therapeutic inquiry to highlight and elaborate a maladaptive interpersonal theme, the therapist concurrently initiates a process of *deconstructing* this theme or life story. A fundamental therapist objective is to help the patient construct a clear and precise picture of the major disruptive interpersonal theme in his or her life. A corollary objective is to call into question the patient's assumptions, expectations, and interpretations about details, situations, and events associated with manifestations of this theme. The therapist scrutinizes the logical consistency and coherence of the patient's stories, throwing a spotlight on the lapses of logic and coherence that inevitably characterize maladaptive interpersonal themes.

Deconstruction of a prepotent maladaptive interpersonal theme interrupts the spontaneous, automatic operation of the underlying dysfunctional internal working model and creates the possibility of perceived new meanings and implications for previously unquestioned interpersonal situations. A large portion of cognitive processing occurs outside of conscious awareness. New situations that contain elements that overlap with plot lines characterizing the content of entrenched cognitive schemas tend to activate these schemas. In turn, these schemas influence the working models of interpersonal interactions that guide behavior (Weston, 1988). A deconstructive dialogue shakes up old patterns of thinking, feeling, and behaving. The possibility is created for new patterns of cognitive processing and interpersonal relating, based on new and more adaptive views of interpersonal experiences (Levenson, 1988). Psychodynamic, cognitive-behavioral, and experiential therapies share assumptions concerning the cardinal importance of (1) revising ingrained, dysfunctional ways of construing life experiences, and (2) creating new, healthier perspectives of one's life. Indeed, such processes of problem reframing succeed, regardless of the domain of inquiry (Schon, 1983).

Years ago there was a popular television show, *Columbo*, about a frumpy homicide detective who appeared to be innocuous and naive. The format for the plot lines never varied: A murder would take place, the audience would know who had committed the murder, the murderer would think the crime was unsolvable, but Lt. Columbo would always solve it. His *modus operandi* was first to gather information, using empathy to understand the suspected murderer's point of view. Then, through repeated observations and questions that appeared naive, he would proceed to progressively pick apart— to deconstruct—the murderer's alibi, which was constructed of inconsistencies, gaps in logic, ambiguities, and falsehoods. Ultimately, when confronted with the tattered remains of what initially appeared to be an airtight story, the murderer would confess that his or her story did not hold up. Of course, the analogy has limits. A therapist ultimately is attempting to help free a patient from confining dysfunction, not arrest a culpable party. The similarity concerns a process of facilitating the patient's realization that the dysfunctional story that has restricted his or her ability to be happy and productive does not hold up under careful scrutiny.

Of course, the inquiry set in motion to achieve this liberating awareness can become adversarial, as it inevitably did in Columbo's investigations. The therapist runs the risk of becoming overly zealous in his or her efforts to help the patient see the errors of his or her ways. What started as a collaborative inquiry can then degenerate into a cross-examination.[1] The deconstructive inquiry also can become adversarial when the patient resists the therapist's efforts to examine uncomfortable issues and to make unpleasant points (Wachtel, 1993). A very common but often undetected situation that contributes to an adversarial inquiry arises when transference–countertransference patterns are enacted amid a hostile interpersonal tone. The therapist's interventions may convey critical, accusatory, or pejorative implications for the patient (Binder & Strupp, 1997a; Henry, Schacht, & Strupp, 1986; Wachtel, 1993; Wiley, 1984). Furthermore, the time pressures associated with brief therapies create unique dangers in this area of therapeutic inquiry. Therapist and patient know that they have a relatively limited period of time in which to work together. This pressure may create a sense of urgency in the therapist to get things done, which can degenerate into impatience with any evidence of resistance by the patient.

Examples of Desconstructive Inquiries

1. A married woman, Joanne, sought psychotherapy because of her inability to decide whether she really wanted to be with her current husband or her previous husband. She portrayed her current husband as reliable about practical matters and exciting but lacking in warmth and empathy. In contrast, Joanne portrayed her ex-husband as unreliable about practical matters but completely devoted to her and their children (who now lived with their mother, the patient). An important part of her tormenting indecisiveness was her view of her ex-husband as genuinely devoted to their children. Unlike her current husband, her ex-husband spent an enormous amount of time with their children, very frequently came over to the patient's house to be with the children, and repeatedly stated that his primary aim was to be

a supportive father. The therapist pointed out certain glaring inconsistencies in this story, which Joanne, although a very smart woman, had glossed over. Although the ex-husband was always ready to run errands with the children, he was habitually late with his child support payments or did not pay them at all. He did spend a great deal of time with the children but often put them in the position of having to choose between doing something fun with him or doing their schoolwork. He stated that his primary concern was the welfare of his children, but he seemed oblivious to the strife created between the patient and her current husband by his intrusions into their home life with the children. As Joanne began to consider these inconsistencies in her ex-husband's behavior, her attraction to him and sense of obligation began to diminish. In this illustration, the therapist was able to (1) draw upon his common-sense knowledge about the appropriate expectations associated with different roles in our society, (2) detect the discrepancies between the picture of the ex-husband's behavior and relevant social role expectations, and (3) point out the logical inconsistencies that were created by those discrepancies in the patient's story.

2. Vanessa sought psychotherapy because of chronic depression associated with feeling unappreciated and unworthy of acceptance and love. The salient maladaptive interpersonal theme in her life was one in which she yearned for intimate, supportive relationships, expected criticism and rebuff for these wishes, tended to misperceive others as critical and rejecting, and pervasively devalued herself. The result was a depressive affect.

After several sessions of weekly therapy, Vanessa began a session by apologizing to her therapist for not being in a good mood. She explained that she had big problems at work with her female boss. The therapist pointed out that Vanessa was apologizing for not being in a good mood with her, a therapist, as if it were expected that she would always be in a good mood when with her therapist. Vanessa acknowledged that since she paid the therapist to listen to her, it should be OK to not be in a good mood sometimes. The therapist then pointed out that even with this rationale, Vanessa still apologized for being in a bad mood. Vanessa finally realized that her assumption about what kinds of moods her therapist would tolerate was irrational. This realization struck an emotional chord, and she then realized how much she always wanted to please others, "no matter what." The therapist observed that Vanessa was making an assumption that pleasing others was accomplished by always presenting a happy face—in essence, by stifling most feelings and hiding them from others.

The therapist proceeded to examine whether Vanessa felt that other people's desire for emotional support from her indicated that they were weak and needy. Vanessa acknowledged that although she saw the desires of others for emotional support as "normal," she assumed that others did not feel the same way about her desires for support. For example, Vanessa assumed that her therapist would be "put off" by any expressions of need or distress, and she feared that any disagreements with her female employer would result in her immediate firing. With further inquiry, however, Vanessa admitted that she had had no experiences with her therapist that would support the assumption that the latter would not tolerate negative affects, and she had no logical reason to believe that her boss would fire her so easily, since she was a good employee with very sought-after skills. The therapist asked whether the image of a critical, ostracizing woman, who was easily annoyed by expressions of need or distress, rang any bells. Vanessa immediately thought of her mother, whom she had spent her entire life trying to placate. In this example, the therapist called into question certain unquestioned assumptions that served as the pillars of Vanessa's conceptual framework for viewing significant relationships. As the deconstructive inquiry led to repeated questioning of these assumptions, Vanessa's view of her possibilities in relationships began to change.

3. Grace was a divorced, middle-aged mother with grown children. She had a successful career but had been socially withdrawn, often isolated, for several years. She never dated and had few friends, even though people often made overtures to spend time with her. She had been married for almost 20 years, but had never felt genuinely in love with her husband. He had been an emotionally cold individual, who grew increasingly disinterested and devaluing toward Grace as the years went on. She eventually initiated the divorce when her children had left home and she felt nothing but emptiness in her marriage. The central issue for Grace was her conviction that other people only valued her for what she could do for them; beyond that they had no desire to be with her. Her most consistent personal contact with other people took place in various self-help support groups that she attended.

Early in therapy she began to have suicidal thoughts associated with a revelation she had had while attending one of these self-help group meetings. Grace concluded that she had sacrificed her life in the futile attempt to please her critical and emotionally rejecting mother. Consequently, her married life had been a waste, because the man she married had been chosen primarily to gain her mother's approval. Her divorced life had been a waste because she was still trying to please her mother, even though her mother was dead. Her therapist responded to this self-revelation by engaging Grace in an examination of the major events in her life. This inquiry revealed that there had been many pleasant experiences in the early years of Grace's marriage, although the relationship had gotten progressively worse in the years just prior to the divorce. In order to compensate for her increasingly unhappy marriage, Grace had become more involved in her work and hobbies, as well as in child rearing. All three of these involvements had yielded impressive accomplishments: children who were personally and professionally successful, a very good career, and beautiful artwork that she had created. The reality of Grace's accomplishments presented major contradictions to her despairing conviction that she had always disappointed her mother, her husband, and anyone else who was important to her, and that all of the sacrifices she had made were for nothing. Her therapist pointed out these contradictions and suggested that the real sacrifice that she had made was her absorption in self-loathing, because over the years it had deprived her of the opportunity to enjoy her many accomplishments. Grace was struck by this observation and began to explore its implications in therapy.

This vignette illustrates a deconstructive inquiry in which a profound life problem is reframed in a way that offered the patient control over her fate. Her framing of the old problem put her fate in the hands of others' judgments, whereas the reframed problem tied her fate to her own self-judgments.

Examples of Missed Opportunities for Deconstructive Inquiries

An old maxim states that reflecting on mistakes can be more instructive than gloating over successes. Likewise, it might prove useful to consider examples of missed opportunities to engage in deconstructive therapeutic inquiries. The examples are drawn from the case of Sidney, the dysthymic man whom we encountered in Chapter 4, who engaged in inconsolable self-loathing and felt trapped in grudging obligations to remain committed to his fiancée and his job. The first example comes from a portion of the treatment in Chapter 4 that illustrated a loss of track of the focal theme. Often losing track of the therapeutic focus goes hand in hand with missed opportunities for a deconstructive inquiry.

A little further than midway through the treatment, the therapist was exploring recollections of family experiences that may have contributed to Sidney's low self-esteem. This topic led to a discussion of past experiences, which the therapist unsuccessfully tried to use to bolster Sidney's self-image. In the process, the therapist missed an opportunity to engage Sidney in a deconstructive inquiry. Again, the interchanges are numbered for clearer referencing.

T1:   Well, what about your mom? How does she figure in all this? Did she have high hopes for you?

Sidney described his mother as being "in awe" of educated people and bitter about her background and lack of education. She had had very high expectations for her son and pressured him to achieve. Although as a child and adolescent, Sidney had striven to meet his mother's expectations, he believed that she had been disappointed in him.

T2:   She wouldn't consider your present position as that of a successful person?

P1:   Well, maybe she would. I guess she would. I mean, she wouldn't know. I guess she just wanted me to be happy, to have all the symptoms of being happy, you know.

T3:   Symptoms? (*Laughs.*)

P2:   Like your job and seem happy, and go to church, and have kids, and just be a well-adjusted citizen.

T4:   Like she was unable to be, but she wanted all that for her son. Would your parents have been in awe of their son, with a master's degree in business?

P3:   No.

T5:   Why is that?

P4:   They were disappointed in me. I guess I was the first one in my family, in all of my family anywhere, to get a college degree.

T6:   And they were disappointed?

P5:   Yes.

T7:   I don't understand.

P6:   Maybe it was because *I* was disappointed. I knew that I didn't have the confidence that I wanted to have when I graduated from college. I can remember when I left high school and thought I was going to college. I said to myself, "God, if I graduate from Central Michigan University in 4 years, I'm going to be confident enough to do anything I want to, so . . . "

T8: And by the time you got there . . .

P7: By the time I graduated, I realized that . . .

T9: It's kind of like you spoil anything you touch.

P8: I should have been able to do much better. I should have been able to graduate at the top of my class if I'd just had more confidence.

T10: Uh-huh.

P9: I feel like a failure. I didn't take any pride at all in graduating.

T11: Was your mother living at the time of your graduation?

P10: Yeah.

T12: Did she come to your graduation?

P11: Yeah. Yeah, they came.

T13: What did she think of all that?

P12: 1 don't know. I don't know. They didn't say much. I didn't see them. We had the ceremony. I'm sure they were proud, but . . .

T14: Did they look around? I mean, this is kind of in your imagination, but would they have sat in the audience and looked around at those other parents? Try to imagine what those other parents were like. Were they doctors and lawyers?

P13: I imagine my parents were intimidated by everything.

T15: Yes. But yet their son was up there graduating, just like everybody else.

P14: Yes.

T16: So they were probably proud of that.

P15: Yes, I would think so.

T17: Proud of you?

P16: Uh.

T18: (*Laughs.*) I know that's pushing it a bit far, but, what happens with all this? It's kind of like you are looking from the outside in, like we just did, trying to imagine what your folks might have felt, sitting at your college graduation. They were proud of you, but when that thought gets right up next to you, it bounces off.

It's almost *impossible* for you to conceive of that, of somebody liking you, or being proud of you, or thinking that you're good. You really resist that thought.

P17: Ah, I don't know what I was going to say.

T19: How do you feel right now?

P18: I'm thinking that after the graduation ceremony, we all went out to dinner. My parents gave me a graduation present, a new pen. But in the move from school, I somehow lost it. I couldn't find it. Both my parents were real mad. And that just shows you right there that I was still the same dummy. I was the same old incompetent that I was when I left 4 years before.

T20: So, those are the people you're trying to please? Whose expectations you're trying to fulfill?

In this vignette there are glaring inconsistencies that signal the influence of a self-created dysfunctional life theme, a manifestation of the CMP described in Chapter 4. Sidney accomplished something unparalleled in his family. He completed college and received a degree and then went on to obtain an MBA. Nevertheless, he was still disappointed in himself and viewed his family as having a similar attitude toward him. The therapist appeared to recognize at least some instances of this pattern but did not pursue them. The therapist directly confronted Sidney (T2) with the question of whether or not his mother would have considered him successful. Sidney grudgingly acknowledged that she probably would (P2), then proceeded to say that she would have wanted him to have all the "symptoms" of being happy. The therapist's response (T3) indicates that he appreciated the implications of Sidney's use of that word to refer to happiness. But the therapist did not pursue an inquiry into why Sidney appeared to be so reluctant to acknowledge having achieved something that he so badly wanted: to make his family proud of him. This was a glaring inconsistency in Sidney's story. Similarly, the therapist did not pursue an inquiry into why Sidney appeared to view happiness over success in life as something abnormal, a *symptom*. This view did not conform to a commonsense notion of happiness.

The therapist initiated an examination of Sidney's recollections of his college graduation day (T11), in an apparent attempt to prove to Sidney that his parents were proud of him and, therefore, that he had reason to be proud of himself. Sidney, however, focused on the loss of a graduation present (P18) as a reason for viewing his college graduation as a disappointment. He ended the story with a strongly demeaning characterization of himself. The therapist responded (T20) with apparent dismay at the reactions of Sidney's relatives. The therapist missed the opportunity to examine another glaring inconsistency that defies commonsense: The accidental loss of a pen was sufficient to spoil a 4-year achievement unparalleled in Sidney's family. How could Sidney consider those two events as comparable by any stretch of the imagination? This question was never asked, and the maladaptive theme that supported Sidney's low self-esteem remained unshaken.

In the penultimate session, Sidney had begun by suggesting that his therapy had been a failure—another failure for which he blamed himself. During the course of the session, his therapist appeared to become exasperated with Sidney's lack of progress and seemed to be trying to cajole Sidney, perhaps somewhat frantically, into some type of constructive action. The therapist suggested that if Sidney had such a dislike for all of the responsibilities associated with his romantic relationship and with his career, he should give them both up and at least take a job he would enjoy until he decided what career he did want to pursue. Sidney's response was to argue that he could give up neither commitment because he had responsibilities. This response was a glaring example of contradictory logic that the therapist did not examine.

In the last session, a discussion ensued about why the therapy had not produced any noticeable change in Sidney's life. Characteristically, Sidney blamed himself, with the explanation that he had not been sufficiently open with the therapist and others. In this discussion a slight inconsistency, with important and relevant implications, appears.

T1: But you seem to connect the idea of being open with the idea of being able to then change, to make change.

P1: To make change.

T2: To make changes. If you can really describe clearly and openly these things, maybe then you could make some changes.

P2: Maybe I can't be open because I don't really know what's bothering me. I don't know, maybe it's just a matter of defining precisely what I feel like needs to be changed. I don't know. Maybe one of the big things that needs to be changed is just to be more open, just all the time. I think that people I work with would like that better. Yeah, they sit around and talk about stereos and DVDs and going to this concert or that concert and not liking this yogurt or chili. I mean, they make an occasion about going out to lunch and talk about what they had to eat. To me, it is a bother just to stop and eat. It's not anything to make a whole production out of. I mean, they enjoy going the whole hour, walking somewhere, sitting and eating and talking about DVDs and the food, and come back talking about DVDs and food.

The ensuing dialogue touches upon issues of shame that are relevant to the patient's focal emotional dynamics. But what is not pursued is the relatively subtle inconsistency having to do with Sidney's supposed dislike for his job and career as a whole. He hates his work, yet it is "a bother just to stop and eat." In this statement he appears to be referring to more than simply finding it uncomfortable to talk with colleagues about personal topics. It sounds as though he is so engrossed in his work that he does not want to be bothered by stopping, even for lunch. On the face of it, this does not seem to be a big matter. Often, however, it is the cumulative impact of examining many small implications of inconsistencies, contradictions, ambiguities, and other narrative gaps that produces a therapeutically significant disruption of a dysfunctional mental working model and corresponding interpersonal pattern. In other words, the cumulative impact of small episodes of deconstructing a prepotent interpersonal theme can lead to major cognitive insight and problem reframing. Conversely, the cumulative impact of many missed opportunities for such a deconstructing inquiry can be failed therapy.

THE IMPORTANCE OF ASKING INCISIVE QUESTIONS

I noted earlier, that any intervention that promotes a good inquiry will contribute to therapeutic change, and that good questions are particularly useful. In traditional psychodynamic therapies the ultimate objective is to identify the hidden meanings of unconscious contents. The primary method for achieving this objective is free association: encouraging the patient to talk in a free-flowing, uncensored fashion, while the therapist listens for evidence of unconscious themes. The working assumption is that unconscious content will be revealed in verbal form through the impetus of drives seeking expression. The therapist searches in relative silence for truths hidden under manifest verbal communications and behavior (Eagle & Wolitzky, 1992; Levenson, 1985).

In contrast, brief dynamic–interpersonal psychotherapy is based on assumptions from interpersonal theory and a constructivist episte-mology. From this vantage point, the person's difficulties are seen as the result of (1) construing personally significant interpersonal events in a particular way that contributes to distress and dysfunction, and (2) continuing to operate interpersonally in a way that contributes to rein-forcing the mental working model that serves as a basis for this way of construing the world. To reiterate: The primary therapeutic objective, then, is to construct as clear and precise a picture as possible of how the person construes his or her interpersonal world and then to de-construct it, in order to identify more potentially rewarding alternative life story lines.

The seminal interpersonal theorist Harry Stack Sullivan (1954) rec-ommended that therapeutic work be based on a "detailed inquiry" to help the patient understand what is going on around him or her, to which he or she is oblivious. Sullivan's primary assumption about the origin and perseverance of psychopathology states that the child be-gins to misread his or her environment because of the psychological conflicts, foibles, and frailties of parental figures, and this proneness to misinterpreting the interpersonal environment becomes increasingly ingrained over time. The dynamic–interpersonal model views dys-functional mental working models and corresponding maladaptive in-terpersonal patterns as the products of this chronic misreading and misinterpretation of interpersonal events. A detailed therapeutic in-quiry is the most effective method of constructing a precise picture of these working models and interpersonal patterns. The anachronistic interpersonal themes are brought into focus, revealing truths that are inherent in manifest content and behavior (Levenson, 1985). To sum-marize this point: How the patient construes the world in ways that produce dysfunction and distress, and how the patient's characteristic transactional patterns reinforce these ways of construing the world, are expeditiously revealed through a detailed inquiry rather than through interpretations of free associations.

Incisive questions are the cornerstone of a detailed therapeutic inquiry. Therapeutic questions are incisive (1) when their content is relevant to the salient interpersonal themes being examined and when they provoke the patient to (2) self-reflect and (3) consider al-ternative ways of perceiving and interpreting thematically relevant issues and other noteworthy problems. During the thematic construc-tion process, incisive questions are an expeditious method of identi-fying and organizing thematic components. During the thematic deconstruction process, incisive questions are an expeditious method of highlighting ambiguities, narrative gaps, contradictions, self-deluding falsehoods, and other forms of illogic. Viewed from a relational perspective, a core feature of psychopathology is the person's oblivion to it; dysfunctional working models and corresponding maladaptive interpersonal patterns are simply taken for granted. The person does not even consider that his or her ways of construing the world and interacting with it are the causes of unhappiness; or, if he or she does consider these factors, they are assumed to be the only alternatives available in the circumstances. Therefore, an incisive question is the most effective technique for engaging the patient in the crucial process of questioning the unquestioned. In order to develop more effective ways of dealing with the world, the patient first has to consider that his or her current methods are problematic and to understand the nature of the problem.

Interpersonally oriented psychodynamic approaches to therapy have appreciated the importance of effective questions, whereas more traditional psychodynamic approaches have continued to assume the primacy of interpretation as a technical change agent. Interpretation is the primary technical intervention when the therapeutic aim is to uncover mental contents defensively hidden from awareness in the unconscious. Interpretation provides the "true" hidden meanings of mental experiences and behavior. If, on the other hand, it is assumed that the patient is not hiding some irrefutable truth but rather has been chronically trapped in an anachronistic, rigidly maintained set of assumptions and expectations about self and the interpersonal world, then an incisive question is the best technical intervention for encouraging the patient to consider alternative vantage points from which to construe the world (Levenson, 1985; Wachtel, 1993). As Wachtel so succinctly put it:

> The difficulties that bring people to therapy derive in large measure from the ways they interpret and give meaning to the events in their lives. Correspondingly, much of what contributes to the resolution of these difficulties involves helping them to create new meanings, to find different ways of making sense of their experiences and, as a result, new possibilities for adaptive action. (p. 185)

The following list summarizes the values of incisive questions:

1. They facilitate patient communications that contain thematically relevant information.
2. They contribute to reframing problem situations in a way that

offers new perspectives and new possibilities for problem resolution.
3. They are a crucial part of modeling and coaching the patient in
   the acquisition of the generic self-reflecting and self-regulating
   skills that are important for problem identification and problem resolution, with or without a therapist's help.
4. They contribute to cognitive insight.
5. They promote therapeutic collaboration and further therapeutic inquiry.

During the course of thematic construction and deconstruction,
incisive questions can serve a number of inquiry functions in addition
to information gathering, such as clarification, confrontation, and interpretation. *Clarification* occurs when a question serves to make more
precise the meaning or nature of a patient's communication. *Confrontation* occurs when a question serves to highlight a contradiction in the
patient's story. *Interpretation* occurs when a question serves to suggest
an alternative meaning to an interpersonal event or self-image that has
hitherto been viewed in a certain way, without question.

Examples of the Therapeutic Functions of Questions

Following are examples of questions that serve different functions, depending on the particular circumstances of the therapeutic inquiry at
the time. These examples are drawn from the seventh session of Carl's
therapy. We encountered Carl, the man who complained of an emotional barrier between himself and others, in Chapters 3 and 4. The
vignette discussed here was examined in Chapter 4 in the context of
illustrating the tracking of a therapeutic focus. We are examining it
again because it clearly illustrates various therapeutic functions of
questions. In the previous session, Carl had focused on his conflicted
relationship with his father, who was portrayed as a highly admired
man who expected a great deal of his children and was bitingly sarcastic when disappointed or annoyed. Carl experienced his father as
being interpersonally very uncomfortable and aloof, and Carl had always wanted a closer relationship with him. In this session, Carl introduced the issue of whether he and his therapist should refer to each
other by first or last names.

P1:   Well, one thing I'd like to start out with is that, um, I don't re-
      ally know how I should address you. Do you have a preference
      for that? I've avoided addressing you because I don't know

how to. (*Chuckles.*) So I usually just say "Hello" and "Good-bye."

T1:   Well, can you say something about your concerns?

P2:   I guess there's two possibilities. I either could call you *Dr. Kaufman*, or I could call you *Charles* or *Chuck*. I guess, I don't know. And I guess maybe I was waiting for a cue from you, but it seems like you don't address me either as Mr. Green or Carl. You just say, "Hello. Wait a minute. I'll be with you in a minute." And then we both just say "good-bye." I guess I thought I should just explicitly bring it up and see if you have a preference or a feeling about it.

T2:   Hmm, why do you think this question is coming up now?

Although on the face of it, Carl's opening question appears reasonable, the therapist is unsure about its implications regarding the focal issue of the therapy, as represented by the CMP. They had not met for 2 weeks because the therapist had been away, which had given Carl time to think about a topic of conversation. The therapist's questions at T1 and T2 represent information-gathering or reconnaissance tactics. He then asked what designation Carl would prefer, who indicated a preference for first names. The therapist asked why.

P3:   I don't know. It seems more informal and relaxed and, uh, friendly.

T3:   Do you feel that last names would be formal and unfriendly?

P4:   (*Laughs.*) Somewhat.

T4:   What would be unfriendly about it?

In this interchange, the therapist's first question (T3) serves a confrontational as well as a clarifying function. Note, also, that this question could be perceived as a bit sarcastic; here the therapist ran the risk of being viewed by Carl as similar to his father in that respect. The question at T4 served a more straightforward and clarifying function.

The therapist eventually told Carl that he preferred to use last names, since they had a professional relationship. Carl assured the therapist that this preference was "OK—I just needed to know what the arrangement would be." Sensing that this topic was loaded with meaning, the therapist probed further for Carl's sentiments. Carl added that the arrangement was appropriate, since the therapist's approach was "pretty analytical." With further probing questions, Carl revealed: "I'm sort of uncomfortable with the whole approach. I always feel a little ill at ease and wishing I could break through that sense of reserve that I get from you." Carl proceeded to complain about the therapist's habit of responding to a question with a question and used the hypothetical question "Well, do you like me?" as an example. Carl further complained that he would "try various things in order to try to unseat you from your attitude. But nothing works." The therapist began to see a parallel between Carl's depiction of his father in the sixth session and his depiction of the therapist in the seventh session. The therapist pointed out Carl's increasing sensitivity to his "reserve." Perhaps in response to the therapist's efforts to prompt Carl to reveal all of his feelings about the name arrangements and about the broader issue of the therapist's relationship with him, Carl expressed his first complaint about the therapist.

P5:   *Uncomfortable* sounds right, but there is something *discomforting* about it too. I have the idea in my mind that since my goal for coming into therapy is to learn something about how to relate to people, and in particular how to become friends with people, that maybe I am feeling that if I am not doing that with you, maybe the therapy isn't really working, or I'm not doing what I came here to do. (*Laughs anxiously.*)

It was difficult for Carl to sustain this openly critical attitude toward his therapist; in fact, he averted a direct confrontation by referring to "the therapy" or "the experience" rather than the therapist. The therapist pointed out that Carl was really complaining about him. In response, Carl admitted that he was particularly bothered by the sense of "reserve."

T5:   What are you dissatisfied with me about? What's missing in my part of the relationship?

P6:   Uh, well, the first thing that occurs to me is just that sense of reserve. Uh, I wish I didn't feel that you had that reserve. So that's the biggest thing that I could come up with. That's what I would say is how I experience your part of it.

T6:   And what about you?

P7:   For my part, I would say that I probably am hanging back and not mentioning things as they come up. I'm letting things develop and not really letting you hook into me.

T7:   Why do you think you are doing that? What do you think holds you back?

P8:   Some kind of risk involved, and I'm not wanting to make waves, and I'm feeling like I'd rather, to an extent, adjust to what your expectations are of the situation.[2]

T8:   Why? Especially since you feel that *you* are dissatisfied with *me*.

Once Carl admitted his discomfort with his therapist's reserve, the therapist asked a series of questions that revealed an interpersonal pattern relevant to Carl's CMP and presenting problem: He was unsure about the therapist's attitude toward him, so he maintained an emotional barrier between himself and the therapist; he was "hanging back," revealing very little of himself. The therapist's questions during this time (T5–T8) highlighted an enactment of the central theme of the therapy and therefore served an interpretive function. His question at T8, the simple interrogative, "Why?", along with a brief explanatory statement, served a confrontational function for the therapeutic inquiry. A few minutes later, the therapist offered a here-and-now transference interpretation (i.e., a metacommunication about the immediate issue between them) in the form of a question.

T9:   If we pull together some of these observations and experiences you have described in the last few minutes, maybe it would help us understand particularly what makes you hold back. You see me as reserved, and you see yourself as holding back because you are not sure what that is about, and you feel a risk, anxious about it. You are also real reluctant to make waves. If you were going to say that you were dissatisfied, you don't want to make it personal. It's hard for you admit that you are dissatisfied with me. Once you did, of course, you said, "It's not only you. It's 50% me." I wonder if you don't read something into my reserve that is, one, I don't like you and, two, that I don't want to be bothered by your feelings, particularly if you've got something to complain about, fuss about, any feelings, whether they are feelings of you wanting to be closer to me or your feelings of dissatisfaction, complaints? So that you feel a need to hold back. Because otherwise I would get mad and be offended, and our relationship would be ruined.

P9:   I think that's true.

This chapter has focused on the basic components of an incisive therapeutic inquiry conducted in brief dynamic–interpersonal psychotherapy. The next chapter continues this discussion of the therapeutic inquiry, with emphasis on the relative importance of inquiring into different areas of the patient's life, including the ongoing therapeutic relationship.

NOTES

1. The degeneration of the therapeutic inquiry into an adversarial struggle is examined in more detail in the next chapter.
2. See Safran and Muran (2000) for a seminal discussion of therapeutic alliance ruptures (discussed more fully in Chapter 7). Carl's indirectness is an example of what Safran and Muran call "avoidance pathways."

6

Competency 4

Planning What to Do and Carrying It Out:
Implementing Change

The last chapter focused on the knowledge and skills involved in establishing and maintaining a productive therapeutic inquiry, leading to cognitive insight. This chapter focuses on how to (1) determine which area of the patient's life will be the most productive place to explore a central therapeutic issue, and (2) facilitate the transformation of cognitive insight into healthier ways of thinking and acting.

THE ROLE OF TRANSFERENCE
AND TRANSFERENCE INTERVENTIONS

Is there a particular area of the patient's interpersonal life that should be the focus of therapeutic inquiry? Throughout most of the history of psychodynamic therapy, one answer has prevailed: Therapeutic change was believed to be greatest when the psychological conflicts and deficits to be modified are experienced with emotional vividness and addressed in the immediacy of the therapeutic relationship. As Freud said: "This struggle . . . is played out almost exclusively in the phenomena of transference. It is on that field that the victory must be won. . . . For when all is said and done, it is impossible to destroy anyone *in absentia or in effigy"* (1912/1958, p. 108). Since Freud wrote these captivating words, a fundamental psychodynamic assumption has prevailed: that salient psychological conflicts and corresponding maladaptive interpersonal patterns will be enacted in the therapeutic relationship. Longstanding intrapsychic conflicts will be unconsciously displaced onto the person of the therapist. Whatever psychological dysfunction impairs a person's life outside of therapy will be replayed, in purer form, within the therapeutic relationship (Greenson & Wexler, 1969).[1]

Through interpretation, the most widely accepted technical strategy for dealing with transference, manifestations of transference are linked to parallel manifestations of these maladaptive interpersonal patterns in outside relationships, and especially to recollections of childhood interactions with parental figures, with whom these patterns were presumed to have originated. By fostering insight into the origin and nature of internal conflict and maladaptive behavior, this "genetic transference interpretation" typically has been considered to be the most powerful conducer of therapeutic change. In his classic psychodynamic therapy text, Karl Menninger (1958) depicted diagrammatically this technical strategy as the "triangle of insight." The triangle stands on its apex, which represents childhood patterns of conflict, and the other two corners represent more recent versions of these patterns, evidenced in current or relatively recent relationships outside therapy and in the relationship with the therapist. The preeminent technical strategy, promoting the most useful insights, is considered to be a series of interpretations that link the three areas in the triangle of insight.

Menninger's guidelines were applied to time-limited psychodynamic psychotherapy by David Malan and his colleagues (Malan, 1976a, 1979) at the Tavistock Clinic in London. Malan renamed the genetic transference interpretation the "transference/parent" (T/P) link, thus emphasizing the side of the triangle of insight that he considered to be of greatest therapeutic value. Malan (1976b) also provided empirical evidence that more frequent T/P linking interpretations were associated with more positive therapeutic outcomes in time-limited dynamic psychotherapy. While Malan clearly assumed that T/P linking interpretations should be used whenever possible, he also recommended that therapists remain responsive to contextual situations: "Once more I must emphasize that no general rule of this kind should be overvalued or taken too literally. Nevertheless the possibility of making the T/P link should always be sought and should be welcomed when it occurs" (Malan, 1979, p. 93). This flexible strategy tends to be employed in contemporary brief treatment models that are based on Malan's approach (e.g., Magnavita, 1997).

From Freud through Malan, a prevailing psychoanalytic assumption was that transference represented the reexperiencing of past conflicted relationships superimposed as distorting templates on current relationships. This conception of transference implies a linear causal impact of psychopathology on the therapeutic relationship; that is, the patient is the source of maladaptive interpersonal transactions within the therapeutic relationship. The therapist's countertransference is a factor only in the event that his or her unresolved psychological conflicts are activated by the patient's transference. Accordingly, there was minimal, if any, discussion of countertransference by the early pioneers of brief dynamic therapy. This situation changed in the late 1970s.

The influential psychoanalytic theorist Merton Gill introduced a radically modified conception of transference that contained interpersonal and constructivist influences (Gill, 1982). Transference was no longer seen as the projection of the patient's internal representational world onto the "blank screen" (i.e., neutral, objective, reserved) of the analyst. It was now conceived of by Gill as part of a dyadic therapeutic interaction in which the therapist is a "participant observer." The patient has certain preexisting interpersonal sets (i.e., rigid expectations about relationships) that influence the way he or she perceives interactions and interprets their meanings. The patient's transference experiences are always "plausible" interpretations of the therapist's behavior and intentions. The experiences constitute transference when (1) the patient's repertoire of possible meanings of interpersonal interactions are severely limited to certain prepotent interpersonal themes, and (2) the patient's behavior tends to evoke reactions in others (i.e., the therapist) that serve to reinforce the patient's rigid expectations (Gill, 1982; Hoffman, 1983). In this view countertransference (i.e., the therapist's personal reactions to the patient's evocative transference enactments) is inextricably entwined with transference.

Transference and countertransference reactions enact a maladaptive interactive scenario that reflects the patient's primary interpersonal problems. This conception is a fundamental part of Wachtel's "cyclical psychodynamics" model of personality and psychotherapy; likewise, it as well, was a foundation for Strupp and Binder's dynamic–interpersonal model of brief therapy (Binder & Strupp, 1991; Strupp & Binder, 1984). From a relational perspective, the therapist's personal characteristics and his or her behavior activate relevant person–situation schemas in the patient that influence the patient's interpersonal working model of their interaction. In turn, the patient's working model influences how he or she construes the therapeutic interaction as well as the transaction patterns enacted, which tend to shape the therapist's behavior in a direction that reinforces the patient's interpersonal working model (Weston, 1988). Maladaptive interpersonal patterns persist

> without ever having been closely examined, these assumptions have been carried forward automatically from earlier phases of the patient's life. The assumptions, and the accompanying attitudes and behavior, persist because the patient unwittingly and self-defeatingly orchestrates significant relationships so as to evoke reactions from others that confirm their fear and assumptions. Thus, interpersonal relationships serve as a vehicle for self-perpetuating vicious cycles. (Strupp & Binder, 1984, p. 137)

In Strupp and Binder's model, accompanying this interactive conception of transference and countertransference was an intervention strategy that placed much less emphasis on T/P links and correspondingly more emphasis on careful examination of immediate patient–therapist transactions. This more emotionally evocative technical strategy had prevailed in the early days of psychoanalysis and had been resuscitated at least once before (Ferenczi & Rank, 1925; Alexander & French, 1946). Influenced by Gill's advocacy of the strategy for open-ended psychoanalytic therapy, Strupp and Binder (1984) applied it to brief dynamic treatment. The strategy was based on three working assumptions:

1. A technical emphasis on T/P linking interpretations carried two significant risks: (a) conveying dismissal of the patient's point of view, or blame, and (b) promoting intellectualization and a shifting of attention away from the most relevant and emotionally engaging material (which was assumed to be found in the immediate patient–therapist transactions).
2. If the origin of all transference enactments is plausible responses to the therapist's perceived actions and intentions, then the interactions of which they are a part should be carefully examined.
3. Transference and countertransference are always intertwined as part of a dyadic interpersonal system and therefore should be studied as a system.

Accordingly, the primary intervention strategy in time-limited dynamic psychotherapy is here-and-now transference interventions or a detailed examination of transference–countertransference patterns. T/P and T/O (i.e., transference/other) linking interventions are made only after evidence indicates that the patient appreciates the influence of the maladaptive interpersonal patterns on the therapeutic relationship; the sole purpose of these linking interventions is to demonstrate the chronic and pervasive nature of the patterns. It was assumed that the primary psychological change process involved emotionally evocative insight into the influence of maladaptive interpersonal patterns while they were being enacted:

> First, the patient must act; then with the help of the therapist, he or she must step back and observe the action; finally the meaning and purpose of the action must be explored. A therapist who is sensitive to the patient's enactments will recognize their emergence and, at appropriate times, freeze the action in order to engage the patient in a rational and dispassionate discussion of what has transpired. (Strupp & Binder, 1984, p. 159)

For most of the history of psychoanalytic therapy, the position that transference analysis (whether applied in the form of T/P Links or a here-and-now strategy) is the cardinal technical strategy was associated with relatively lengthy treatments. From the 1960s through the 1980s transference analysis was applied in brief dynamically oriented therapies without significant modifications. Whereas traditionalists did not believe that transference would have time to develop in brief treatments, most of the developers of these treatments assumed that the influence of transference was always present and that the focus of brief therapies should be the most salient transference patterns (Malan, 1976a; Davanloo, 1980; Luborsky, 1984; Strupp & Binder, 1984). However, these brief dynamic therapists held assumptions about therapeutic process and change that were developed during their formative years doing long-term psychoanalytic therapy. Patients and therapists made extended commitments of time and emotional engagement to relationships that involved multiple meetings per week for years. These relationships obviously became of paramount importance. In extended, emotionally intimate relationships, which patients were encouraged to view as the center of their lives for the duration of the treatments, it is small wonder that transferences (and countertransferences) flourished.[2]

With accumulating clinical experience conducting brief therapies during the 1990s, I grew increasingly skeptical of this position concerning the cardinal role of transference and transference analysis. I noticed that even with a mind-set geared to identify and examine here-and-now transference–countertransference patterns, the therapeutic inquiry primarily addressed relationships outside of therapy in a very high proportion of the time-limited therapies that I conducted.[3] Maladaptive interpersonal patterns were routinely identified in current and past relationships, leading back to childhood recollections and establishing a pervasive maladaptive influence.

Subsequent to Malan's (1976b) demonstration of a positive association between frequency of T/P linking interpretations and positive outcome in brief dynamic therapy, empirical studies of the role of transference interpretations have not supported its exalted role in this form of treatment. Employing improved methodology (e.g., using session transcripts instead of therapist process notes taken from memory; blind raters), Marziali (1984) was not able to demonstrate as clear-cut an association as did Malan. Two other independent research teams have found no relationship between type of intervention, including transference interpretations, and outcome in brief dynamic therapies (Crits-Christoph, Cooper, & Luborsky, 1988; Silberschatz et al., 1986). Both teams did find, however, a positive association between the content relevance of interventions to an identified therapeutic problem focus and positive outcome. In other words, it appears that the particular issues focused on have more bearing on treatment outcome than the specific types of interventions used and the areas of the patient's life in which these issues are explored. A more recent study, utilizing more precise methods for tracking salient interpersonal themes in the therapeutic relationship and outside of therapy, has reported that in a majority of patients the major problematic interpersonal issues addressed in outside relationships are not detected in the therapeutic relationship (i.e., there is no evidence of relevant transference enactments) (Connolly et al., 1996).

In the late 1990s, two independent research teams that have been studying the relationship between transference interpretations and outcome in brief dynamic therapies for over a decade came to the same conclusion: Patients with relatively mature interpersonal functioning may benefit from low-to-moderate levels of transference interpretations (i.e., not more than one or two per session, at most). Patients with relatively less mature interpersonal functioning may benefit from zero-to-low levels of transference interpretations (Connolly et al., 1999;

Ogrodniczuk, Piper, Joyce, & McCallum, 1999). In other words, based on the most convincing research to date, the consensus is that transference interpretations may be beneficial *in low doses*, but the use of transference interpretations in brief dynamic therapy does not appear to be essential. Another researcher, who has also conducted extensive investigations of the role of transference interpretations, summarized this point succinctly:

> Interpretations of the here-and-now transference manifestations are potentially potent and accurate. But the relationship with the therapist may seem unimportant to the patient compared to the interpersonal difficulties outside of therapy. (Hoglend, 1996, p. 129)

Recently Hoglend (2003) reviewed all of the empirical investigations over the last decade of the relationship between use of transference analysis and outcome in brief dynamic therapy, including his own substantial body of work. He concluded:

> A moderate use of transference interpretation may be more productive with subgroups of patients [receptive patients with high levels of interpersonal relating]. However, it may be sufficient, *or even more important* to focus on interpersonal relationships outside therapy. (p. 286, emphasis added)

Why does there appear to be such an enormous discrepancy between the prevailing psychoanalytic "wisdom" regarding the role of transference interpretations and the empirical evidence, at least as this wisdom is applied to time-limited dynamic therapies? As noted, traditionally for patients in psychodynamic treatment, if the therapeutic relationship were not the single most important relationship in their lives, it was at least very psychologically significant. This state of affairs is understandable for a lengthy, time-consuming (multiple times per week) relationship in an epoch when a relationship with one's doctor had strong paternal overtones.[4] Until the late 1980s, the doctor–patient relationship in the U.S. health care system was stable and nurtured over time. The psychotherapy relationship was part of this system.

This all changed in the last decade of the 20th century with the rise of "managed care" in this country. Doctors no longer care for patients; now, health care providers deliver a service to clients or consumers, and this service is strictly regulated by an impersonal monitoring system. The role of the health care provider is to assist in the resolution of circumscribed problems as efficiently and rapidly as possible. The doctor–patient relationship tends to be highly transient. Doctors have little time to spend with individual patients. Furthermore, employers are continually changing insurance plans in the never-ending struggle to minimize rising premiums, which requires patients to seek new doctors because the old ones are not covered under the new plans.

Psychotherapy and therapist–patient relationships are part of this system and reflect the value put on efficiency and problem solving. Psychotherapy relationships tend to be relatively transient and focused on circumscribed problems. Consequently, there often is less emotional attachment on the part of either patient or therapist. The relationship does not have the same psychological significance for the patient as it did during the previous health care epoch. It could be argued, then, that the typical time-limited therapeutic relationship may not be the same prepotent magnet for transference enactments that it was in lengthier treatments during an epoch when the therapeutic relationship occupied a more prominent role in the patient's life.

It is also true that the theoretical frameworks of open-ended relational treatments are relatively more cognitive and interpersonal, and the technical strategies are more oriented toward resolving the contemporary real-life versions of patients' problems. Interpretive links are more likely to be made for evidence of salient themes across sessions, regardless of the area of the patient's life in which they appear (e.g., Frank, 1999; Wachtel, 1993). This strategy is characteristic of "expert" therapists in brief dynamic therapies, who emphasize work on relevant problems in real-life relationships (Connolly, Crits-Christoph, Shappell, Barber, & Luborsky, 1998; Goldfried, Raue, & Castonguay, 1998).

In sum, there is converging clinical and empirical evidence suggesting that a transference-focused technical strategy is no longer warranted in time-limited dynamic therapies. *Instead, the most frequent area examined in detecting the influence of dysfunctional internal models of interpersonal relationships and corresponding maladaptive interpersonal patterns is that of relationships currently significant to the patient. Furthermore, the most frequent type of linking interpretation is one that draws parallels between maladaptive interpersonal patterns in the patient's current relationships and reconstructions of problematic childhood relationships with significant parental figures.*

I do not mean to imply that transference interventions should be avoided altogether. I believe that when skillfully implemented, they can have enormous therapeutic impact. A constructive transference intervention requires a precise combination of factors: the right time, succinct language, and a nonpejorative mind-set. After conducting an intensive examination of the role of transference interpretations in one therapy, Gabbard and his colleagues (Gabbard et al., 1994) put it well: transference is a "high-risk, high-gain phenomenon" (p. 59). As a general rule, I would recommend that transference interventions be used when either of two conditions exist[5]:

1. The therapist identifies evidence of transference–countertransference patterns reflecting the maladaptive interpersonal themes that are the focus of treatment, and the patient evidences a receptivity to examining these patterns.
2. The therapeutic alliance is significantly strained, indicating that transference–countertransference enactments have reached a critical threshold of influence.[6]

I have discussed the topic of transference at length for two reasons. First, as already noted, the technical strategy of transference analysis has prevailed in both long-term and brief psychodynamic treatment approaches, including the approach that I helped develop over 20 years ago (Strupp & Binder, 1984). Therefore, I think it is important to review this position as well as the reasons for my departure from it. Second, I still believe that in brief dynamic–interpersonal psychotherapy, transference interventions can have a profound therapeutic impact at certain times and when delivered competently.

An Example of Transference Analysis

A segment from the therapy with Carl was described earlier in Chapter 5. To recap: Carl felt uncomfortable and out of place with people because he experienced an "emotional barrier" between himself and others. Carl held himself back from others because he assumed that they would view his desire for closeness as selfish and unappealing. Several sessions into the treatment, he had begun with the issue of what he and his therapist should call each other. Their discussion quickly revealed that the underlying issue was a variation of the central issue of the treatment: namely, that Carl wanted a more personal relationship with the therapist but assumed that he would be rebuffed. Consequently, he was wary of exposing his feelings and held back. The therapist pointed out this pattern with a transference intervention in the form of a question (see p. 164). Carl agreed.

P: I think that's true. And I think that maybe I'm waiting for you to indicate the appropriate level of closeness in our relationship.

T: So if you're waiting for me to sanction how close and how open you can be with me, and I don't do that, then you hold back. But it's still based on the assumption, for you emotionally, that unless I give you tangible assurance that I like you and that I want to hear you, your conclusion is that I don't like you and I don't want to be disturbed by you, by your emotional life.

P: Well, I don't think that intellectually, but that is my sense of it and what I have been acting on.

Carl proceeded to obfuscate the issue temporarily with an intellectualized discourse on how deferring to others' presumed preferences for interpersonal closeness is generally the way social interactions work. His therapist dealt with this defensive retreat with a series of mildly confrontational questions concerning this supposed guideline. This portion of the therapeutic inquiry established that Carl's adherence to this guideline is associated with his holding himself back from others and with his interpersonal discomfort.

T: It sounds like you follow that guideline . . .

P: (*Laughs.*)

T: . . . of social intercourse, and it leaves you feeling dissatisfied and people close to you dissatisfied. So maybe another way to put the first question is, "Where did that guideline come from?"

P: (*long pause*) My father would have to be that source. (*pause*)

The therapist's interpretive and confrontational questions have prepared Carl to make an interpretation for himself that links an important facet of his central issue to the three major areas of his life: outside significant relationships, the therapeutic relationship, and the relationship with his father. The immediate context presents an opportunity for a T/P linking interpretation: Carl's guideline about social interactions, which dictates his way of relating to the therapist, is based on his relationship with his father. The therapist encouraged Carl to continue.[7]

T: Can you elaborate?

P: I think both in his actions and his reactions, my father doesn't tell you about things that he is uncomfortable with. On the contrary, he'll withdraw if he's uncomfortable. And in his reactions, if he senses that you are coming to him with something that you're uncomfortable with, he'll also withdraw. I guess that I picked up from those behaviors that that is the way to behave, both because it's a good way to get along with him, and also because that's the way he behaves.

T: I was wondering about that, too. It sounded a lot like the way you described your father and your relationship with him. It makes me wonder if the way you experienced your relationship with him—the way you interpreted his emotional distance—is the prototype for other relationships. Maybe he is not interested in you or doesn't even like you. By not even liking you, I mean, look, you're growing up, you're a little kid, and here you have this imposing figure, your father. You're bursting with all kinds of things that you want to tell him, reactions that you want from him. And he doesn't seem to want to listen to you or give anything back. What conclusion can you draw? The obvious conclusion a kid would draw is that he doesn't want to be bothered with you, doesn't even like you. You're not worth the bother. What I'm suggesting is more than just speculation, because look at what you experienced with me today. You have described me as "reserved," and that must mean that I don't want to be bothered by your feelings, and maybe I don't even like you.

The immediate relevance of a rather lengthy T/P linking interpretation, including a good deal of speculation about Carl's formative childhood experiences with his father, is buttressed by referring back to what has recently transpired between Carl and his therapist (Strupp & Binder, 1984). Carl's construal of what is permissible in the relationship with his therapist is based on his experiences with his father. A therapeutic inquiry that is hitting the mark—that is, touching the patient in a personal way and resonating with his or her conscious and unconscious experiences—is often indicated by the patient's expanded view of his or her inner life, including an enhanced emotional experience (see next section).

P: Yeah. I'd go along with that. You know, since we last talked, I have been trying to recall more experiences about my childhood: what it was like, places that we lived, and what my father was like. What kind of relationship did I have with him? And I couldn't come up with anything. Then sometime during the week I had a dream about a man I had worked for in one of my first jobs out of college. He treated me so nice and was so supportive and approachable. I remember in the dream that it made me feel so warm, so good, the way he treated me, so opposite of my father. In the dream I remember that he took such a concern with how I was doing, it made me feel like crying. This man seemed to care about me more than my, my—*gosh*—I just blocked on the word *father*.

This memory and its meaning was so emotionally loaded that Carl momentarily forgot the much-used word *father*. The therapist pointed this out, and Carl explained that he thought it reflected his ambivalence over speaking critically about his father. The therapist inquired about the deep feeling exposed in the dream. Carl reported that it was an experience for which Carl still longed. The therapist then inquired about Carl's immediate response to these memories.

T: As you're recalling it, does it stir up any feelings now?

P: Yeah, it is somewhat the same feeling of wishing that I could have a relationship like that and also be a person like that or just have that quality. I think, in some ways, the man in the dream represents what is lacking in my life.

T: Is there any of the feeling right now?

P: Yes, though just when I started describing it, I lost a bit of it, but if I think about it—if I just think about his face as I imagine the dream—I can bring up that feeling. It's like a feeling of longing that I have to go back years to have fulfilled.

T: You know, even as you're feeling some of it now, from the outside, you're very successful at keeping it well hidden inside.

The therapist comments on Carl's unemotional demeanor as he talks about a profoundly emotional experience.

P: I'm sorry. I am not being real successful at getting into it.

T: Even as you said, even as you start talking about it, it fades.

P: Mm-hm.

T: Which is kind of striking, because, you know, just as often, if not more typically, as you talk about feelings they become clearer. In the context of what we've been talking about today, I wonder if there's a part of you that feels that even as we're talking about assumptions regarding what you can share with other people, maybe you're not being fair to yourself or to them—in this case, me—because you're still very much operating under those assumptions. As you begin to talk about feelings with me, there's a part of you that feels you have to stifle them, that I don't want to be burdened with them.

P: I don't know if that's it or not, but I do know that this feels like it's a very deep thing. And it's very hard for me to stay in touch with it because of that. As you were talking, I started to get more in touch, and now as I start talking, I'm losing it again.

T: As though you can't share it. You know, if that's what's happening—if you begin to get closer to sharing these very personal feelings with me and then feel you've got to stifle them—it is such a contrast to that dream in which you so much want to be close to and to share feelings with a man, your first boss . . .

P: Mm-hm.

T: . . . your father, me. I mean, you had the dream shortly before we were going to meet again, and that's what you began with today. It sounds like you very much want us to be closer, but the more directly we talk about it, the more the feeling fades.

P: (*Sighs*) Mm-hm.

T: By the way, there is also something that I think would be very important to look for in other relationships: The more you want to be closer to somebody, the more the feeling of it gets stifled—with your wife, your child, other people.

P: (*long pause*) All I can say is "*yeah!*" I know, I feel a bit dumbstruck by how much your view resonates for me.

The therapist made a here-and-now transference interpretation about a maladaptive pattern enactment (i.e., stifling feelings when discussing an emotionally loaded topic), reflecting the therapy's central issue, as it was actually transpiring between them. This intervention illustrates the consummate therapist skill of reflection-in-action, whereby the therapist is able to "freeze the action" to comment on the immediate process or to adjust his or her actions in response to the immediate contextual circumstances (Schon, 1983). Metacommunication about the therapeutic interaction is the most experientially vivid way of examining relevant dysfunctional working models and corresponding maladaptive interpersonal patterns (Safran & Muran, 2000; Strupp & Binder, 1984). When implemented skillfully (i.e., stated clearly and succinctly, at a time when the patient is receptive to hearing it, and with a nonpejorative interpersonal tone), this type of intervention can be a powerful facilitator of cognitive insight. It can also elicit a therapeutically beneficial emotional experience by (1) encouraging the patient to accept previously "strangulated" (or in other ways, pathologically managed) emotions, and (2) by experiencing the liberating feeling that often is associated with gaining perspective on dysfunctional ways of construing interpersonal reality and maladaptive patterns of interacting in which the person has been immersed, sometimes for a very long time. In this example, Carl gained access to previously hidden longings and sadness; eventually he was flabbergasted by his role in creating a barrier between himself and others because of his discomfort with these longings for interpersonal closeness.

THE THERAPEUTIC ROLE OF INQUIRING ABOUT EMOTIONS

In the preceding vignette, the therapeutic inquiry led Carl to the realization that he had strong longings for closeness and a deep sadness over his failure to attain that closeness with important people in his life. Yet, he had only fleeting direct experiences of these emotions. A cardinal characteristic of psychodynamic psychotherapies is the fundamental role ascribed to emotions in producing therapeutic change. Early psychoanalytic theories of psychotherapy advocated simple release or catharsis of "strangulated affects" as the primary curative process (Freud, 1893–1895/1955). This view initially was applied to brief psychodynamic psychotherapies in the form of "unlocking" pent-up unconscious urges and affects (Davanloo, 1980). More contemporary psychodynamic theories view the identification, acknowledgment, and acceptance of disturbing, hidden emotions as part of a process of modifying defensive and adaptive personality structures to facilitate more constructive management of psychic life and interpersonal relations (Magnavita, 1997; McCullough-Vaillant, 1997). It matters little whether acceptance of a previously disavowed emotion (e.g., anger, guilt, sadness, shame) is viewed as leading to more adaptive compromise formations or a more mature and harmonious internal representational world. The point of agreement is that emotions associated with conflict or general dysfunction must be acknowledged and accepted in order for healthier functioning to occur.

Prevailing psychoanalytic "wisdom" also posits that understanding one's conflicts leads to change only if it is accompanied by vivid reexperiences of the emotions associated with the psychic issue being revealed and understood. In brief dynamic therapies this presumption is reflected, for example, in the strategy of "unlocking the unconscious" (Davanloo, 1980; Della Selva, 1996) as well as in the strategy of reexperiencing maladaptive interpersonal patterns at the very time that the patterns are being analyzed through the transference (Strupp & Binder, 1984). There is some empirical support for the change-inducing function of emotional arousal during therapeutic inquiry (McCullough & Andrews, 2001). On the other hand, there is also ample empirical support for the effectiveness of cognitive-behavioral therapies with a wide variety of disorders and problems, and this approach tends to deemphasize explicit inquiry into and experiencing of emotions (Hollon & Beck, 2004).

A resolution to this apparent contradiction can be found in the information about the person contained in the emotions. Although emotions do have physiological and subjective components not found with cognitions, emotions and cognitions share certain important adaptive functions. Both phenomena provide information about the status of the psyche and about the status of the individual's relationships with significant others. Furthermore, within the rich experience of emotions, there often is an important "story" about issues that are at the heart of the individual's psychological world (Urist, 2000; Wiser & Arnow, 2001). Both cognitions and emotions are part of the individual's information-processing activities, and both acquire their current meanings from the immediate interpersonal context. In other words, issues around the acknowledgment, expression, and acceptance of emotions always have either explicit or implicit interpersonal consequences and/or implications. I propose that the fundamental mutative element in emotional expression is the disruption of previously rigidified internal working models and corresponding maladaptive interpersonal patterns. Furthermore, I propose that this process of creating a disequilibrium could be as effectively activated by disrupting either previously ingrained cognitions *or* interpersonal patterns. It is an individual matter.

In my clinical experience cognitive understanding and emotional awareness tend to blend together. Furthermore, people vary greatly in their characteristic propensity for being aware of and willing to experience their feelings, as well as in their openness and demonstrativeness in expressing emotions. The management of emotions is part of a person's character style, which is unlikely to change greatly, even in long-term treatment. Certainly, in brief therapy there is neither the time nor (typically) the inclination to even attempt to change a basic characteristic such as style of emotional management. However, the management of certain emotions may be considered pathological or maladaptive because of the irrational interpersonal implications associated with the emotions: for example, squelching anger because the emotion is presumed to be harmful to others, or squelching sadness because it is presumed to be a sign of weakness that will put off important others. In such circumstances, it may feel liberating to finally ventilate such feelings, if such open expression is within the person's capabilities. But what is really necessary is to understand and change the interpersonal meanings and implications of the emotions in question, whether or not the emotions are fully experienced. Such a goal is within the striking distance of brief therapy processes.

I do believe that there is a certain type of emotional arousal that is necessary for significant therapeutic change to occur in time-limited therapy. This arousal represents a mix of sentiments, including discomfort in current circumstances, trust and hope in the therapy relationship, and curiosity about the targets of the therapeutic inquiry. Finally, there is excitement and a sense of liberation associated with discovering a new perspective during the therapeutic inquiry, a new way of comprehending things that promises to make a difference in one's life and future. This type of emotional arousal accompanies an engrossing meeting of the minds, in which patient and therapist realize they have constructed an important shared understanding. The patient may feel a sense of liberation and the therapist may feel exhilarated in response to being on the "same wavelength." This shared experience is what the humanistic clinicians call "meeting" the other person (Bohart, O'Hara, & Leitner, 1988).

Examples of Emotionally Engaging Therapeutic Work

1. Howard, whom we met in Chapter 5, felt greatly relieved when he realized that his intensely negative reactions to his new stepson were provoked by the similarity between the behavior of his stepson and his ex-wife. Up to this point, Howard was unaware of making

the connection. Once pointed out, however, he was astonished that the similarities were so obvious and that he had been so consciously oblivious of them.

2. The work with Carl, previously described, concerning the relationship implications of using first versus last names illustrates intensely personal emotions that have been squelched (in this case, sadness associated with a longing for closeness with his father). The segment of therapeutic inquiry described earlier in this chapter also illustrates the sense of liberation associated with seeing something very important about oneself for the first time with vivid clarity. In this case, Carl comprehended how his fear of others being put off by his feelings, particularly his desire for closeness, caused him to squelch those desires along with the sadness associated with the absence of genuine intimacy. He was "dumbstruck" by this insight. The emotions experienced by Carl were produced during a segment of transference analysis characteristic of time-limited dynamic psychotherapy (Strupp & Binder, 1984). In the following two illustrations, important interpersonal patterns are identified that lead to emotional arousal, but not within the patient–therapeutic relationship.

3. Norman, who first sought psychotherapy to deal with work issues, wanted to deal with his social isolation after those issues dissipated. The central issue in CMP terms was that Norman wished to receive understanding and support from significant others but expected to be ridiculed and rebuffed for those desires. He tended to misperceive overtures by others as inevitably leading to intrusiveness and criticism, and he responded with proactive irascibility as well as emotional and interpersonal withdrawal. His withdrawal left him feeling inept and worthless. Earlier examples of the therapeutic inquiry had focused on his apprehension over asking a woman from his book club for a date. He had anticipated that the other members of the club would laugh at him. When he finally made a date with the woman, Evelyn, he became very stressed by the assumption that he would have to entertain her every minute. As they explored this experience (see Chapter 5, pp. 146–148), Norman began to realize the irrationality of his assumptions and to see the chronic maladaptive pattern from which they derived. First, the therapist tried to unearth evidence of the central issue's influence on the therapeutic relationship, but Norman did not admit to any such experience.

T: In regard to this experience of feeling like you've got to live up to the expectations of the other person, or entertain the person in some way, or that you're going to be judged about whether you're interesting enough to have a relationship with, do you ever feel any of that with me, in our relationship?

P: No.

T: That you're being judged by me and that you have to act or be a certain way?

P: Not exactly like that. I know that you're making judgments, and I know that they're professional judgments, and it's like it helps you to help me.

T: Well, the kind of judgment I was talking about, if I've been hearing you right—the kind of judgment you've been experiencing or anticipating—is whether or not you're worth being around or worth having a relationship with.

P: You know, I have been thinking about this issue, and I realized that it applies not only to my relationship with Evelyn but to any face-to-face relationship. I'll get thoughts, you know, like "What do these people really think of me? How am I coming across to them?"

T: Yes, well, I guess that was one of the implications of the connection with work—that if you don't meet their expectations, they'll fire you.

P: Yes. I'm not so focused on that now. I'm not so much concerned by my task performance, but more about myself interpersonally: How do they perceive me as a person? Do they think I'm just a dumb shit? I mean, not that I don't know the details of my job, but that I don't have the common sense that an adult should have.

T: What if they thought of you that way? What did you imagine the consequence would be?

P: They would be making a mental judgment that there is something lacking in me. The one word that comes to mind is *stupid*.

T: *Stupid*. Does that word bring to mind anything?

P: Yeah. It's a verbal insult that I remember getting from my father for doing stupid things, in his estimation.

T: Like what?

P: I guess the one that's most memorable would be trying to help him around the house, fixing things, and so forth. He always yelled at me for things like not picking out the right tools to give him.

T: So, just being a kid, just having the foibles of a kid is enough to be seen as stupid.

P: Yes.

T: That's when he was hard as nails.

P: Exactly!

T: But that real stern, judgmental, hard-as-nails drill sergeant dad is still having an impact on you in your recollection of him.

P: Yes.

T: You expect your colleagues at work or a woman on a date to act like a drill sergeant.

P: No. I don't expect them to be hard like that. But I will do anything in my power not to be perceived as dumb or stupid, and at different times during my life, I have felt that way.

T: But it's kind of like a default setting for you, isn't it? That you have to work hard not to be seen as stupid. I'm trying to put into words what I think you're describing as your experience. It's not accurate, but it's like your experience. It's like you are continually in danger of being in that position, and you have to struggle and work constantly not to be seen in that way. It's the default position.

P: Yeah. Yeah. Yeah. I reacted to that.

The therapist helped Norman connect this pattern of anticipating ridicule for his desires and efforts from his coworkers and romantic partners to his father. These nontransference-related connections were very meaningful for Norman. His resonance with them produced the sense of liberation mentioned, as well as a very personal affective experience.

T: What does it bring up?

P: Well, it just sounds so true. I mean, I didn't get any thoughts as a result of it, but it's like, just the words you used—it's just so true, just hearing that.

T: Does it bring up any feelings?

P: What?

T: Does it bring up any feelings?

P: Just sadness. I mean the fact that it is true. It makes me sad that it is true. Because that's obviously not a good thing, but it's right and I try not to get into that position again but, you know, every now and then it does happen.

Norman described how he had gone to work after graduating from high school, because his grades were not good enough to get into college. He attributed his poor academic performance to an "I-don't-care" attitude that originated with his parents, who appeared not to care.

P: Well, it's easy for me to say that nobody motivated me. Neither of my parents provided any encouragement to do well in school or to go to college.

T: Before we got into this discussion, that sad feeling emerged immediately around your picture of yourself struggling to avoid this default position of being stupid that is associated with your father calling you stupid. Then we started looking at the sadness this other issue from your childhood, your family, brings up, and which you've talked about before: not feeling that your mother or father invested a whole lot into the matter of guiding you. They sort of just let you kind of hang out there.

P: Right.

T: I wonder if that's an important source of sadness: feeling like they just didn't seem interested enough to care about what the hell you were doing?

P: It could well be a very significant part of it. Yeah. I always enjoyed being around my friends and their families, more than I enjoyed being with my own family. I don't know if that is typical of kids or not.

T: Well, that's common, but it can have very different reasons.

P: When I was with my friends and their families, I felt that was better. That would make me envious, but I suppose that could make me sad, too. You really have struck a nerve with this—I mean, at least going back to that time when I was a kid.

The anticipation of ridicule and rebuff from his parents when wanting understanding and support and the feeling that they had no interest in guiding and mentoring him were related issues for Norman, to which he and his therapist had traced connections from current relationships to recollections of familiar family patterns. This inquiry was associated with the emergence of a chronic sadness in Norman, whose defensive squelching of it during his life had contributed to his problematic traits of irascibility and social withdrawal.

4. Michelle, in her late teens, sought psychotherapy to understand why she had tried to commit suicide with an overdose of prescription medication. The suicide attempt had taken place in her first year of college. After the attempt, she had spent several days in a psychiatric hospital and then had returned home to recuperate. Michelle was currently living with her mother, stepfather, and younger sibling. Her parents had divorced when she was a small child. She had continued to have regular contact with her father until several years after he had remarried and had another child. She had not spoken to her father for several years. Michelle did not get along with her stepfather, who was portrayed as a crude, highly critical individual, about whom her mother continually complained. Michelle had always had a circle of close male and female friends who were especially important to her, because she avoided any romantic attachment. She was convinced that a boyfriend would inevitably hurt her.

After Michelle's suicide attempt, her mother had encouraged her to live at home rather than returning to school, so that she (her mother) could provide emotional support. When Michelle returned home, however, she found that her mother was gone most of the time, leaving Michelle to care for her younger sibling. It was evident that this situation reflected a role in the family that Michelle had played prior to going to college and into which she once again was recruited: to be a good girl, who tried unsuccessfully to please her highly critical stepfather and to rescue her mother from a stressful marriage.

Michelle described how after she left for college, her mother would call her almost daily to complain about her miserable marriage, tacitly imploring Michelle to make her feel better. Michelle was doing well at school and enjoying herself. However, she began to feel increasingly guilty, helpless, and overwhelmed—feelings that culminated in her suicide attempt.

After the brief hospital stay and her return home, Michelle began to have increasing contact with her friends; she also planned activities for the summer and made plans to return to college at the beginning of the fall semester. She described, however, numerous arguments with her mother over these activities. Mother disapproved of her phone calls with friends, of her trips with friends away from home, and of her desire to return to school. Mother argued that Michelle needed to rest, recuperate, and spend time with her family.

Michelle's relationship with her male therapist would be best characterized as a subtly idealized paternal transference, with her therapist sensing a pull from Michelle to take care of her. Earlier in Michelle's treatment, her therapist had offered the following interpretation: Her mother was emotionally drowning in her conflicted marriage, and like a drowning person, she was thrashing about for someone to whom she could cling for support. Although overtly claiming to care for her daughter, tacitly the mother was desperately clinging to Michelle for emotional support, and she was frightened and resentful of Michelle's relationships with friends and plans to leave home again.

Michelle responded to this view of her family situation as if a door to a dark, confining room had been thrown wide open. She experienced the first sense of exhilarating liberation from the feelings of guilt and helplessness that had weighted her down. As time went on, she initiated contact with her father. It turned out that he and his family were glad for the renewed relationship with Michelle. In addition, for the first time Michelle began a romantic relationship with a young man with whom she had been friends for a while. The changes initiated by Michelle appeared to result from a liberating new perspective of her family dynamics rather than any significant release of pathologically managed emotions.

TRANSFORMING INSIGHT INTO BEHAVIORAL CHANGE: PRACTICE AND COACHING

An especially satisfying experience for psychodynamically oriented therapists is the attainment of new understanding about some portion of the patient's problem. Therapist and patient agree that they have achieved an important insight about dysfunctional thinking (*perhaps* including recovery of previously unconscious issues) and maladaptive patterns of interacting. An unfortunately common and disconcerting aftermath of such an experience is the bafflement often felt by the therapist when the patient asks, "But what can I do to change?" The therapist is stumped, because traditional psychodynamic theories of psychotherapy have not adequately addressed this eminently practical question. Psychoanalytic drive/structural theory posits that making unconscious conflictive mental content conscious, especially as the content is manifested as transference, will conduce change.[8] Psychodynamic object relations, interpersonal, and relational theories posit that new "corrective" interpersonal experiences, particularly within the therapeutic relationship, are primarily responsible for change. A strategy of here-and-now transference–countertransference analysis, or, synonymously, "metacommunicating" about the status of the therapeutic relationship, along with the therapist's provision of a healthy interpersonal relationship, is considered to be the most effective method for conducing change. Modern brief psychodynamic treatment models are frequently based on this conception of change (see Levenson, 1995; Safran & Muran, 2000; Strupp & Binder, 1984).[9]

All of these theories assume that change in mental processes and corresponding interpersonal patterns of relating occur spontaneously as a product of insight, particularly when transference enactments are involved (i.e., acting out conflicts within the therapeutic relationship) or when new interpersonal experiences occur within the therapeutic relationship (e.g., when the patient, arriving late for a session, expects to be criticized for doing wrong, as he has been by significant others throughout his life, and the therapist does not do so). But there is no convincing body of evidence for this assumption. From a conceptual standpoint, the idea of insight spontaneously conducing change leaves the crucial change process too haphazard and uncharted. Furthermore, even if change could be produced by the internalization of "corrective" experiences within the therapeutic relationship, questions arise about whether those experiences will actually transpire, and if they do, whether sufficient time will be available for the internalizations to take hold and conduce lasting change. These questions are particularly germane to brief therapy, where the time available for therapeutic experiences is relatively short. There also is the issue, raised above, concerning the frequency with which therapeutic relationships in brief therapy are psychologically important enough to the patient to carry the primary responsibility (and sufficient valence) for conducing change.

Modern theorists have questioned the hegemony of experiences within the therapeutic relationship, involving either insight or internalization, as conducers of change. This trend was begun by Alexander and French (1946), who saw corrective interpersonal experiences in real life as more therapeutically mutative than experiences in the "shadow play of life" represented by the therapeutic relationship. Some contemporary relational and theoretically integrative theorists have taken the position that whatever transpires during the patient–therapist collaboration must be overtly and directly applied to life outside of therapy for change to be truly meaningful (Frank, 1999; Wachtel, 1993). For example, Wachtel (1993) states: " . . . The contemporary emphasis on the analysis of transference and on the mutative properties of the relationship per se places too great a burden on what transpires in the consulting room" (p. 62). Later in the same book, Wachtel continues the point: "Much of the process of change in psychotherapy . . . takes place outside of the therapy sessions. For meaningful therapeutic change to occur, the patient must apply his insights in his daily interactions with others" (p. 256). Occasionally the observation has been made that the therapeutic relationship, whether in intensive analytic therapy or brief dynamic therapy, represents a small portion of the patient's life, and that other significant figures and experiences will have more impact (Hoglend, 2003; Wachtel, 1993).

Insights and experiences attained within the therapeutic relationship may indeed be mutative. Nevertheless, for all the reasons given previously, the focus of brief dynamic–interpersonal psychotherapy should be on the patient's relationships in the outside world and on helping the patient develop interpersonal skills that will allow him or her to continue the work on his or her own. Acquisition of these interpersonal skills represents a positive therapeutic change, and they are very unlikely to be acquired spontaneously; rather, active and directive interventions by the therapist are required. The notion of the dynamic therapist having a role as interpersonal coach and mentor, as well as interpreter of mental processes, has always been a current in psychodynamic thinking. Often, this view was implicitly reflected in therapeutic strategies that advocated active measures for dealing with neurotic problems. For example, Ferenczi and Rank (1925), whose views influenced later psychodynamic brief therapy pioneers, encouraged their patients to take specific, concrete actions to deal with neurotic inhibitions. Several decades later, Alexander and French (1946), whose work also inspired contemporary brief psychodynamic therapists, continued the call for active, willful changes in interpersonal behavior as a follow-up to insight. Contemporary relational and dynamically oriented (but theoretically integrative and technically eclectic) theorists, representing both long-term and brief treatment approaches, have advocated incorporating more active strategies and techniques into treatment, including cognitive-behavioral techniques (Frank, 1999; Magnavita, 1997; Wachtel, 1993).

The point is this: The dynamic–interpersonal brief therapist functions as a coach and mentor around life issues, particularly interpersonal issues. As is true for any coach, teaching and facilitating the use of certain skills are the ultimate goals. In the case of brief dynamic–interpersonal therapy, the skills in question are first and foremost certain generic interpersonal skills. These skills were introduced in

Chapter 2 and are considered necessary to facilitate therapeutic change processes. They include:

1. Interpersonal pattern recognition is a semiotic skill involving the identification and recognition of meanings associated with verbal communications, and recognizing meanings and themes embedded, often subtly, within interpersonal interactions.
2. Self-observation is the skill of being able to reflect upon and appraise one's own mental processes, experiences, and behavior associated with interpersonal interactions. Self-monitoring is the corollary skill of extending the act of self-observation over time.
3. Reflection-on-action involves the use of self-observation to critique one's interpersonal behavior after the behavior has occurred, in order to improve future interpersonal performance. Reflection-in-action involves using self-observation to appraise and modify one's behavior *as it is occurring*, thereby creating enormous flexibility that fosters the capacity to improvise in initiating and responding to interpersonal behavior. Reflection-in-action is the quintessential feature of expertise in any performance domain (Schon, 1983).

Attainment of these skills in the domain of interpersonal relations is a major therapeutic achievement. They equip the patient with resources that can be used to deal effectively with life's challenges and problems long after therapy has ended. Other psychodynamically oriented clinicians have recognized the significant therapeutic potential of generic self-observation skills. For example, Fonagy, Steele, and Steele (1995) have stated:

> The treatment . . . enhances the development of reflective self-function and may, in the long run, enhance the psychic resilience of individuals in a generic way and provide them with improved control over their systems of representations of relationships. The development of this function equips them with a kind of *self-righting capacity* in which, through being able to operate on their internal working model, the latter can become an object of review and change. (p. 267, emphasis added)

The specific "coping skills" that are typically referred to in the therapeutic literature, particularly the brief treatment literature, are relevant for dealing with particular issues, situations, or interpersonal circumstances. In contrast, the generic skills enumerated here comprise the foundation upon which any interpersonally-related coping skills are based. The patient is able to use them to comprehend the nuances of interpersonal interactions in any situation.

Any performance skills, including these generic interpersonal skills, are most effectively taught in the context of real-life problem situations, rather than in an abstract format (Bransford, Franks, Vye, & Sherwood, 1989). In brief dynamic–interpersonal psychotherapy, this means examining interpersonal episodes from the patient's life that can be used to progressively elaborate, clarify, and sustain a precise working model of the central interpersonal issue of the treatment. The generic interpersonal skills are necessary to construct and then deconstruct interpersonal themes, with the purpose of short-circuiting and modifying the dysfunctional mental processes and corresponding maladaptive interpersonal patterns in which these themes are manifested.

All of the major forms of psychotherapy have coaching strategies that, at least implicitly, foster the acquisition of these generic interpersonal skills. Cognitive-behavioral psychotherapists use journaling, rehearsal, and structured homework assignments between sessions. Gestalt therapists use role playing, the "empty-chair" technique, and detailed metacommunications about the patient's immediate experiences. Psychodynamically oriented therapists tend to be the most circumspect about their coaching strategies, because their theories of psychotherapy characteristically proscribe active, directive interventions. Nevertheless, effective dynamic therapists tend to coach their patients in the acquisition of generic interpersonal skills through subtle questions and comments about the patients' life experiences that have subtle structuring or suggestive elements (Wachtel, 1993).

Psychodynamically oriented therapists characteristically believe that the therapist's role should be limited to helping the patient make his or her own choices about any course of action. The therapist should not impose his or her own values and attempt to influence the patient's behavior. However, avoiding the use of any influence or persuasion is likely to result in no impact at all. The therapist who restricts him- or herself to dispassionate observation and interpretation is not likely to effect change. In psychodynamic theory this passive role traditionally has been presumed to foster patient autonomy. I propose, however, that autonomy is most likely to be attained through the acquisition of skills that enhance the person's effectiveness in dealing with life's challenges. Insights, even deeply felt ones, produce only a foundation of declarative knowledge. Such knowledge remains inactive unless it is translated into useful actions at appropriate times; in other words, it must be translated into procedural knowledge. This translation is not likely to take place spontaneously. It needs the impetus produced by effective and directive therapeutic coaching.

The most common coaching strategy used by brief dynamic–interpersonal therapists focuses first on identifying, with the patient, a central issue in the form of a dysfunctional interpersonal working model and corresponding maladaptive interpersonal pattern. Next, the therapist explicitly encourages the patient to (1) look for evidence of this central issue in life experiences (particularly interpersonal encounters), (2) "freeze the action" (i.e., catch oneself in the maladaptive act), (3) consider healthier alternatives, and (4) act differently. The therapist explicitly encourages the patient to engage in retroactive self-monitoring or reflection-on-action, as well as encouraging ongoing self-monitoring reflection-in-action and behavioral modification during an episode of maladaptive action.[10]

An example of this kind of coaching is taken from the treatment of Norman, whose case has been discussed previously. The current segment comes from the session discussed in Chapter 5, in which Norman was struggling with his inhibitions around asking a woman for a date, because he feared that any overtures would be rebuffed.

T: Now you said you don't want to [ask Evelyn for a date] because it hurts to be rejected, to have someone say "no." That is understandable. But do you feel that is a particularly significant situation for you?

P: Yes. Especially if it is public, because then I am sort of subject to ridicule.

T: By whom?

P: Nobody, in particular. But it's, umm . . .

T: You just assume you are going to be ridiculed?

P: Yes.

T: For what?

P: I guess for something that would be construed as, ah, an embarrassment or a failure. Some feeling like that.

T: So if you are at a social event at church and ask a woman if she would like to dance, and she says "no," . . .

P: ... I would be completely embarrassed and anyone seeing this would laugh at me.

T: Why do you suppose the woman would be sure to say "no," and why are you so sure that anybody seeing this would laugh?

P: Because I would have failed somehow.

T: It appears that you assume that everyone would have the same attitude as your dad had—they would be mocking, sarcastic, and caustic.

P: Yes, something like that.

T: We know that your father discouraged the expression of feelings, and neither of your parents was demonstrative in his or her expressions of love. They just did not show love. In addition, your father was sarcastic and made fun of anyone who showed feelings. It seems that this situation gets transposed onto current situations, like the one you imagine at the church social.

P: (*The patient continues to look sad.*) What can I do about it?

T: The main features of that old situation get transposed onto current situations with adults. So when you want closeness or acceptance, you assume that inevitably you will be rebuffed by a woman and other adults will laugh. They will be laughing at someone who is vulnerable and a failure.

P: But how can I change that?

T: The first step is to recognize when it is happening. Practice catching yourself being influenced by these old assumptions. But in order to practice this, you have to put yourself in situations where this old pattern can occur.

P: I know.

The Therapeutic Importance of Practice

The coaching process illustrated in the above therapeutic interaction is repeated throughout brief dynamic–interpersonal treatment. In traditional psychodynamic terms, coaching refers to "working through" the central issue. Interpersonal skill acquisition requires *practice*, the bedrock of any skillful performance. If therapeutic change is conceived as the development or enhancement of generic interpersonal skills, particularly around a central issue, then the primary means of achieving this change is through practice in using these skills. The therapeutic techniques characterizing the different therapy models (enumerated above) all represent forms of practice. In my previous text on time-limited dynamic psychotherapy (Strupp & Binder, 1984), practice was implied in the primary technical strategy of here-and-now transference–countertransference analysis. In time-limited dynamic psychotherapy practice occurs in the form of *in vivo* examination of the central issue, as manifested in the therapeutic relationship. This strategy is effective when the central issue is, in fact, manifested in the patient–therapist relationship, and the patient is receptive to examining it. As previously discussed, however, both of these conditions do not occur with sufficient frequency in today's brief therapies. Furthermore, the time-limited dynamic psychotherapy model was based on the psychodynamic theories of the time, in which therapeutic change was presumed to occur as a product of cognitive insight into salient, conflicted interpersonal patterns combined with internalizations of new relational experiences with a benign therapist. The acquisition of generic interpersonal skills through *in vivo* practice was not sufficiently appreciated.

In brief dynamic–interpersonal psychotherapy, interpersonal experiences outside of the therapeutic relationship are the patient's primary focus for practicing generic interpersonal skills (acquired in sessions) to deal with manifestations of the central issue of the treatment.[11] The therapist guides or coaches the patient in the development and refinement of these skills during discussions with the patient before and after the designated interpersonal experiences.[12] As mentioned above, *in vivo* coaching of the patient in learning to skillfully manage interpersonal interactions, particularly around the central issue, can be an effective strategy when transference enactments of the central issue are detected and when the patient is receptive to examining them. This form of coaching involves here-and-now transference analysis (or metacommunicating) along with explicit guidance on how to reflect-in-action, such as what questions to ask oneself in order to gain a perspective on transactions in which one is currently immersed. Metacommunication about the influence of the central issue on the therapeutic relationship is absolutely necessary during therapeutic alliance ruptures. This occurrence is discussed in more detail in Chapter 7.

Therapeutic coaching involves more than guidance in the acquisition and refinement of generic interpersonal skills. Often the patient must be helped to articulate healthier courses of action. This help might include, for instance, specific suggestions on a course of action or several alternatives. Although traditional psychodynamic theories of psychotherapy eschew such directiveness, the fact remains that patients often need help in learning life skills that may have been arrested due to chronic avoidance of certain kinds of interpersonal situations (Wachtel, 1993). The therapist's role inherently involves persuasion; the patient is most likely to preserve and strengthen his or her autonomy by improving his or her life skills. To briefly reiterate: Interpretive work done around transference–countertransference patterns and recollections of childhood relationships can be applied to the task of understanding and clarifying the dysfunctional interpersonal working models and corresponding maladaptive patterns of relating that are influencing current outside relationships. Connections made between transference enactments and outside relationships are especially effective in convincing the patient of the omnipresence of the central issue. It is likely that examining outside relationships for evidence of maladaptive interpersonal patterns is the most common approach in modern brief dynamic therapies. Explaining the central issue as a vicious interpersonal cycle (Strupp & Binder, 1984; Wachtel, 1993) provides a comprehensible reason for its persistence. Connections made between evidence of the central issue in recollected childhood relationships and current outside relationships serve to create a plausible and meaningful story—that is, narrative understanding—about the origin of the central issue.

CONSOLIDATING THERAPEUTIC EXPERIENCES: INTERNALIZATION

The internalization of corrective interpersonal experiences as a change process in brief dynamic psychotherapy traditionally has been viewed as a product of transference–countertransference analysis in which the therapist is the primary good object (Strupp & Binder, 1984). In dynamic–interpersonal psychotherapy, the primary therapeutic change process involves therapist and patient working together to identify a central issue in the form a dysfunctional mental model of interpersonal relations and a corresponding maladaptive pattern of interpersonal relating; then the therapist coaches the patient on how to replace this mental model and corresponding interpersonal interaction pattern with healthier versions of each. In this case, the internalization of corrective interpersonal experiences occurs primarily in the context of lived relationships outside of treatment. The patient practices the generic interpersonal skills that he or she has learned about in psychotherapy to modify his or her interpersonal behavior outside of therapy. As the patient construes interpersonal experience differently and acts accordingly, other people tend to react in a manner congruent with the patient's new interpersonal actions. The results are benign cycles of complimentary interpersonal behaviors that provide repeated corrective experiences that are internalized.

The cumulative impact of internalizing the corrective interpersonal experiences that occur in outside relationships hopefully serves to consolidate the new mental models and corresponding adaptive interpersonal patterns that the patient has been attempting to implement. Since brief psychotherapy provides very limited opportunity for internalizing corrective interpersonal experiences within the therapeutic relationship, the process I have been describing is especially important for this form of treatment. Practice applying generic interpersonal skills to the central therapeutic issue and practice trying out healthier forms of relating, guided by therapist feedback, hopefully prepares the patient to continue the practice and resulting interpersonal skill development after therapy ends.

Internalization of corrective interpersonal experiences through the therapeutic relationship *does* occur in brief dynamic–interpersonal psychotherapy. In a general sense, it is the inevitable product of a strong therapeutic alliance and successful collaborative patient–therapist relationship. When transference enactments noticeably shape the therapeutic relationship, internalizations will occur to the extent that the therapist limits his or her recruitment into countertransference roles (Levenson, 1995; Strupp & Binder, 1984). Finally, internalizations occur as a product of successfully resolving ruptures in the therapeutic alliance (Safran & Muran, 2000). This process, which involves skillful management by the therapist, is the topic of the next chapter.

TREATING SPECIFIC SYMPTOMS OR PROBLEMS

A patient in psychoanalytic psychotherapy asked her therapist about her diagnosis. He replied that she was a "human being." This diagnosis carries the potential for substantial problems and for impressive achievements. The conceptual viewpoint associated with offering this diagnosis is characteristic of the seminal models of psychodynamic, cognitive-behavioral, and humanistic therapies. Specific symptom pictures and manifest life problems reflect broader intrapsychic and interpersonal dysfunctions that can be effectively addressed using the generic technical principles and strategies that define the specific treatment model. It matters little which treatment model is used. As mentioned, they all are more or less comparably effective.

On the other hand, as described in Chapter 1, a view currently in vogue contends that mental disorders are optimally treated by matching specific symptom syndromes or behavior problems with treatment protocols that have been found to be the most effective empirically with those syndromes or problems (Chambless & Hollon, 1998). A more recent middle position is offered by treatment manuals that specify technical strategies based on patient characteristics but leave the therapist free to use whatever techniques are preferred, as long as they are consonant with the empirically dictated strategy (Beutler & Harwood, 2000; Piper et al., 2002).

As yet, there is no clear-cut empirical evidence supporting the superiority of any of these positions. Relative influence is a function primarily of professional politics and the outside influence of policies originating from public and private treatment reimbursing sources. Given these circumstances, the brief dynamic–interpersonal therapist is on reasonable ground in taking the position that most mental/ interpersonal disorders can be effectively addressed using the generic technical principles described in this book. At the same time, the therapist's effectiveness can only be enhanced by learning specific research-based techniques to address specific symptoms and behavior problems. Amelioration of specific symptoms and behavior problems by the use of specific techniques can, at least, serve to provide the patient with hope, emotional "breathing room" to work on more generic issues, and strengthen the therapeutic alliance. Such techniques can be found in the many technique-oriented treatment manuals available.

The use of a circumscribed protocol to treat specific symptoms or problems, however, is comparable to a physician treating manifest physical symptoms without addressing underlying causes and lifestyle contributions to the symptoms. I propose that reducing the probability of relapse or development of other problems is most effectively achieved by providing the patient with some insight into his or her salient dysfunctional mental models of interpersonal relations, along with practice in detecting and modifying the maladaptive interpersonal patterns associated with these mental models. Perhaps most important, I propose that patients are in the most solid position at the end of therapy if they have become familiar with, and begun practicing, the generic interpersonal skills that underlie all manifest attempts at ameliorating specific symptoms and problems.

A WORD ON SELF-DISCLOSURE

In relational forms of psychodynamic psychotherapy the therapeutic interaction increasingly is conceived from the vantage point of partici-pant-observation and intersubjectivity. Patient and therapist are en-twined in a dyadic system characterized by reciprocal influences (Frank, 1999; Levenson, 1995; Strupp & Binder, 1984; Wachtel, 1993). The therapist's role has evolved from that of a dispassionate observer and interpreter, to a benign object offering a corrective experience to internalize, to a real person (having evident foibles and idiosyncrasies) with whom the patient must learn to deal in a more adaptive fashion than has occurred in previous significant relationships. Along with this view of the therapeutic relationship and the therapist's role is an in-creasing tolerance for, and even encouragement of, prudent self-disclosure by the therapist to further the therapeutic work (Frank, 1999; Leven-son, 1995; Strupp & Binder, 1984; Wachtel, 1993).

Furthering the therapeutic work through therapist self-disclosure has been described most commonly as revealing the therapist's per-sonal (i.e., countertransference) reactions to the patient's maladaptive modes of interacting in a narrowly focused way. The aim is to help the patient understand and appreciate how his or her impact on others serves to reinforce and perpetuate maladaptive interpersonal patterns. A related context for self-disclosure arises when the therapist is experi-encing positive, or at least dispassionate, sentiments and intentions to-ward the patient and reveals these to highlight the contrast between the therapist's actual experience and the negative assumptions held by the patient about the therapist's private experience of him or her. In this case, the therapeutic aim is to spotlight the dysfunctional interper-sonal working model guiding the patient in his or her interpersonal re-lations.

Another form of self-disclosure that is less frequently discussed involves using personal and professional experiences to help persuade the patient of the validity of a point that the therapist is making. This strategy is consistent with the conception of the therapist as a thera-peutic coach whose aim is not only to foster understanding but also to facilitate application of that understanding in real-world actions—in essence to guide and encourage the patient in learning more effective interpersonal skills. For example, the therapist might share personal experiences about him- or herself, unspecified family members, per-sonal acquaintances, or unspecified patients to illustrate how other people cope with issues similar to the patients. Likewise, these unidentified people might be alluded to as exemplars of how problems similar to the patient's can be overcome. It has been suggested that experienced therapists tend to find increasingly diverse therapeutic uses for self-disclosure (Frank, 1999). I believe this inclination reflects not only the value placed on participant-observation as a therapeutic process but also the gradual evolution of the therapist's role, with cumulative experience, from one of technician to one of mentor. I have more to say about this notion in the Epilogue.

Judiciously applied therapist self-disclosure can be used as a form of psychoeducation as well as to deal with problems that arise in the therapeutic relationship, particularly around transference–countertransference issues. Competence in the management of the therapeutic relationship, in order to establish and maintain a therapeutic alliance, is the subject of the next chapter.

NOTES

1. This phenomenon is even more likely to take place in the standard psychoanalytic situation, because the patient is reclined and unable to see the analyst; therefore, fantasies about him or her will have more influence.
2. In the conduct of psychoanalysis and open-ended psychodynamic therapy, a standard practice was to inform the patient that he or she would have to take vacations at the same time the therapist took time off for vacation. Patients routinely accepted this rule. The therapeutic relationship was *that* important. It is unlikely that patients in today's typical brief therapies would accept this rule.
3. There is some, at least, indirect empirical support for this anecdotal observation (Crits-Christoph, Demorest, Muenz, & Baranackie, 1994).
4. From the 1960s through the early 1980s, when the practice of open-ended psychodynamic therapy probably reached its peak, doctors were seen as fatherly figures who were very much a part of their patients' lives and were devoted to caring for them. Older readers may recall the television character "Marcus Welby, MD," a kindly figure who ministered to the same family members for years. In stark contrast are the rushed and highly stressed doctors in the popular medical television show at the beginning of the 21st century, *ER*. These doctors may form brief intense relationships with their patients, but they do not have time for the kind of stable relationships that are psychologically significant over an extended period of time.
5. Based on a review of relevant research, including the extensive research programs led by William Piper, Ogrodniczuk and Piper (1999) recommend

that the following conditions be met for effective use of transference interpretations: (a) the therapeutic relationship is characterized by a strong alliance; (b) supportive interventions are used frequently to maintain the alliance; (c) the patient has "moderately good" capacity for mature object relations; and (d) the patient has evidenced a receptivity to work with transference. In essence, the therapy has to be going well for transference interventions to work. In contrast, Safran and Muran (2000) advocate the use of transference interventions in the form of "metacommunications" when the therapeutic relationship is in trouble. This position is discussed in more detail in Chapter 7.

6. The emergence of therapeutic alliance strains and ruptures is discussed in Chapter 7.

7. This interchange was first described in Chapter 3 to illustrate the hypothetical reconstruction of childhood events, in order to provide a hypothetical origin to current maladaptive interpersonal patterns.

8. Brief therapy models based on this view include the pioneering works of Davanloo (1980), Malan (1976a), and Sifneos (1979). Contemporary models are represented by Magnavita (1997).

9. Although Levenson's brief therapy model is similar to that of Strupp and Binder's, her experience has also led her to the conclusion that the "supply of [transference] interpretations far exceeds the demand," and that patients need more direct coaching than formal presentations of psychodynamic theory recognize. Consequently, her current approach is closer to the model presented here than to the original Strupp and Binder model (personal communication, November 24, 2003).

10. *Action* here refers to covert mental acts as well as overt behavior.

11. See Crits-Christoph (1998) for a summary of empirical evidence supporting this claim.

12. A relatively new area of empirical investigation is that of the patient's mental representation of the therapist, which serves to guide the patient's behavior between therapy sessions (Orlinsky & Geller, 1993).

7

Competency 5

Relationship Management

A therapeutic inquiry is productive only if the patient is motivated to participate in it, regardless of the emotional discomfort that may be involved. This motivation comes from the patient's experience of the therapist as someone to be trusted and liked. In other words, productive therapeutic work occurs only in the context of a strong *therapeutic alliance*. The patient's experience of a strong alliance with the therapist is the best predictor of a positive therapeutic outcome (Horvath & Greenberg, 1994). There also is evidence that a strong therapeutic alliance early in therapy is particularly important to the outcome of treatment (Horvath, 2001).

Recommendations to therapists about cultivating a therapeutic alliance emphasize the importance of conveying certain qualities, including warmth, interest, empathy, respect, and sensitivity to differences in attitudes, values, and interpersonal expectations associated with cultural, ethnic, racial, and gender differences (Strupp & Binder, 1984). There is no question that a strong therapeutic alliance rests on the quality of a therapist's involvement with his or her patient. People seek psychotherapy because they are unhappy or dissatisfied with their lives. In one way or another, they are not able to function adequately or are not able to meet their emotional needs in their interpersonal relationships. The problems that patients experience in their important relationships sometimes significantly affect their therapeutic relationships, and therapists are pulled unwittingly into patterns of unproductive interactions. Hostile interactions between patient and therapist, often very subtle, frequently go undetected; even if they are detected, therapists have an extraordinarily difficult time in managing them effectively (Binder & Strupp, 1997a). And yet, there is empirical evidence that early alliance problems can be overcome if therapists detect the problems and have the skills to deal with them (Foreman & Marmar, 1985; Lansford, 1986; Suh, O'Malley, & Strupp, 1986; Horvath, 2001; Safran & Muran, 2000).

From a dynamic–interpersonal perspective, strains and ruptures in a therapeutic alliance reflect the influence of prepotent transference and countertransference enactments (Binder & Strupp, 1984; Safran & Muran, 2000). A question of great relevance for designing therapeutic technical strategies concerns the prevalence of such transference–countertransference enactments in brief dynamic–interpersonal therapy. In other words, is it inevitable that an alliance rupture in the form of a transference–countertransference enactment will have a significant impact on a therapeutic relationship in brief dynamic–interpersonal therapy? I do not think so.

In support of this opinion, several studies have failed to demonstrate that the same maladaptive interpersonal pattern associated with a patient's troubles is present as a transference pattern in a majority of the therapies studied (Barber, Foltz, De Rubeis, & Landis, 2002; Connolly, Crits-Christoph, Barber, & Luborsky, 2000; Connolly et al., 1996). Connolly et al. (2000) concluded: "Although interpretation of transference to the therapist might be a particularly powerful therapeutic tool, in a short-term focused psychotherapy transference may not be sufficiently developed in the therapeutic material for some patients to warrant the use of transference interpretations" (p. 369).

In my current version of brief dynamic–interpersonal therapy, I advocate dealing with the erratic nature of central maladaptive interpersonal patterns by examining and striving to change them in whatever current relationships they manifest themselves. I assume that patients can learn interpersonal self-awareness skills retrospectively, with a therapist, by reviewing recent interpersonal transactions that occurred outside of therapy, and then subsequently practicing what has been learned in nontherapy relationships.[1] Actually, the therapist's interventions should focus on a central maladaptive interpersonal theme *wherever* it is manifested (see Crits-Christoph & Connolly-Gibbons, 2001).

THE DYNAMICS OF RESISTANCE

To reiterate the conception of therapeutic process developed in Chapter 2, my current working assumption is that, while not inevitable, therapeutic alliance ruptures in the form of salient transference–countertransference enactments may occur. If such an enactment reaches a threshold of strength sufficient to cause an alliance rupture, it must be addressed. It is likely that a transference–countertransference pattern with that much influence will reflect the central issue that was associated with the patient seeking treatment.[2]

From a dynamic–interpersonal perspective, *alliance ruptures* and *transference–countertransference enactments* are assumed to be synonymous. From this same perspective, both terms also contain the more general concept of *resistance*. In contrast to the traditional psychoanalytic notion of resistance as an intrapsychic event that involves the operation of impersonal defense mechanisms working against the therapist's objectives, a dynamic–interpersonal view refers to the nature of the interaction in which the patient and therapist are participating. For example, Strupp and Binder (1984) viewed resistance as "... unconsciously derived personal actions aimed at maintaining a sense of security and avoiding some form of danger, and directed by unconsciously held convictions about oneself and others" (pp. 181–182). A therapeutic interaction can be characterized as resistant when one or both of the participants are caught up, unwittingly and unreflectively, in an enactment of a transference–countertransference pattern.

Resistance represents a strain or rupture in the therapeutic alliance. Such a rupture can be manifested as an overt transference–countertransference enactment. For example, early in therapy, a patient who expected people on whom she relied to be omniscient (like a small child's idealized version of parents) complained to her therapist, "I can't believe the questions you are asking me are so dumb!" An exploration of the patient's dissatisfaction quickly revealed that she expected people who truly cared about her to know what she was thinking. More frequently—and insidiously—alliance ruptures are manifested as covert transference–countertransference enactments. In these cases, clues to the enactment can be detected in disguised allusions to the therapeutic relationship, embedded in the content of whatever the patient is discussing. For example, a patient's complaints that her mechanic is too vague about what is wrong with her car may also refer to her dissatisfaction with her therapist for not being sufficiently forthcoming about what he thinks about her. Such disguised allusions also may be embedded in the meanings of the transactional patterns that currently characterize the therapeutic relationship (Safran & Muran, 2000; Strupp & Binder, 1984). For example, a pattern of interrupting each other before the person talking has finished develops between a therapist and patient. Such a pattern may reflect a tacit struggle for control of the relationship.

An Illustration of Alliance Ruptures

The following vignettes are taken from early and later sessions of a brief psychotherapy that foundered badly when an early covert alliance problem was not detected until it had grown into an overt alliance rupture. Sarah, a single woman in her late 20s, sought psychotherapy for the first time because she was depressed over her inability to maintain a satisfying romantic relationship with a man. Although she was an intelligent and attractive woman, none of her romantic relationships had lasted very long. Either Sarah or the man with whom she was involved at the time would eventually break off contact because the relationship did not develop any depth. When Sarah was between relationships, she felt unattractive and unlovable; when she was dating someone, however, she quickly began to experience any growing interest by the man as undermining her autonomy. If he wanted to spend more time with her, she felt stifled and drew back. Sarah's mother was admitted to a mental hospital for an extended period when Sarah was a teenager. Rather than providing the emotional support that she and her young siblings needed, her father had pulled Sarah into the role of surrogate mother for the other children. It is easy to see that Sarah may have carried burdensome feelings of abandonment, mistrust, and resentment toward men. At the beginning of an early session of treatment, Sarah alluded to a short business trip she had taken with her father. She worked in his business and expected to take it over someday.

P: I don't know what to talk about, because I was real busy since I met with you last week. I went out of town Sunday with my father, and I just got back yesterday.

T: I see.

P: So I was just real busy with business and didn't really have that much time to concentrate or think about what you asked me to think about.

Apparently, the therapist had suggested that Sarah think about certain issues that they had discussed during the last session. Evidently, she did not comply.

T: So you've been really . . . Your time has been taken up. Was this a business trip?

P: Yes.

T: How is that for you, working with your father and working on business things with him?

Notice that with her opening statement, Sarah had tacitly invited the therapist to determine the topic of discussion. Her therapist seemed to accept the invitation and suggested what appeared to be a relevant topic: the recent business trip with her father. Her subsequent communications, however, suggested that a central issue around autonomy struggles with her father was also being enacted very subtly with her therapist.

P: Well, it was nice this past weekend, because we left Sunday and came back late Tuesday night. We were together, probably, for a longer time then we have been in many years.

T: Is that right?

P: It was the first time that I have taken a trip with him out of town for a long time.

T: I see.

P: It's been a long time. And since it was business related, we talked to each other about business, which is all he can talk about. So, if I can meet him on that level, then I can talk with him. But if I can't meet him on that level, then nothing happens.

T: Nothing, like a personal . . .

P: Right, right. So, from the minute I went over to his house and got into the car with him and rode to the airport until I came back—business. And it really got to me on the plane coming back. Just all of the sudden, it hit me about halfway here, that I could not talk about business anymore. All of a sudden, I became so tired that it was all I could do to walk off the plane and get my bags. I just . . .

T: It sounds like it just drained you.

P: It did, because he just kept on and on. At that point on the airplane, I had taken a magazine and I was starting to look at it, but he just kept on and on. I reached a point when I thought, "I just want to look a this magazine. I don't want to talk. I don't want to talk about business!" But he was still all keyed up and . . . sometimes I want to get away from it. But I find myself having really gotten caught up in it, because it's basically the only thing I really have in my life that I can say "This is mine." And someday it could all be mine.

T: So, there's like two sides to it for you. One, you get tired, it drains you and you'd like to get free. But then it's also a very important thing.

Sarah went on to describe how she and her father encountered a business associate on the plane ride home, and in the ensuing discussion, her father had stated how important Sarah's support in his business was to him. Sarah told her therapist that although she appreciated the employment security provided by her father, she often felt that she had no choice in the matter. She originally had planned on going to college. But her mother had been hospitalized just prior to Sarah's graduation from high school. Her father was emotionally devastated by his wife's hospitalization, so Sarah chose to forgo college and work for her father, primarily to provide him with emotional support.

It can hardly be a coincidence that after covertly inviting the therapist to determine the topic of conversation, Sarah had proceeded to express her sense of helplessness and frustration with her father's dominating the conversation on the way back from the business trip. This theme was further complicated by her conflict over feeling obligated to support her father and her own sense of undermined autonomy. She felt that in order to please him and show appreciation for what he had given her, she must stifle her own wants. Is this the prototype for her expectation of any close relationship with a man? More immediately, is this the scenario that has been set in motion in the therapeutic relationship? This issue had not been identified by her therapist, at least not as an influence in their relationship, and by the last third of the planned brief therapy, Sarah expressed strong dissatisfaction with the therapist and therapy.

P: So, what are you thinking about this case now?

T: About this case? Does this feel like a review time for you? What's leading you to have that question?

P: Because I just don't think anything can be done. I don't have, I just really don't . . .

T: How are you finding yourself feeling about that?

P: This is just really difficult at times. It really is.

T: It's difficult? Can you say something about that? In what way is it difficult for you?

P: Just everything. I just don't think there is anything that can be done, except for me to somehow just keep finding the strength to keep going on, just hoping that someday things are going to be different for me and that I'm going to reach a point where things will fall into place and I will be happy.

T: Yes.

P: I just have to hope things are going to get better. I just have to wait

T: And so the difficult part, in terms of this work, is connected with what? What is it about this work that is real difficult?

P: It just seems so pointless.

T: Yes?

P: And I don't mean to say that, but I don't think there's value in this for me. I just don't think there's any guidelines here that can help me. I really don't.

T: Yes?

P: I really don't. It's just the way things are.

T: Yes?

P: I just have to someway be able to keep coping with it, like I have been doing the past few years.

T: Yes. I would think that would be leaving you with some feelings about the work here. It's a disappointment or frustration.

P: It's frustrating.

T: Frustration. Yes.

P: It is, because I don't know from talking with you what can be done, because basically I just see that there is nothing. I think my biggest problem is that I don't have any hope.

T: Yes?

P: I don't . . .

T: Would you think, then, that's one of the things that influences what can happen in here, that hopelessness?

P: I think it does, because I think I'm somebody who came in here without any hope of anything getting any better anyway.

T: Yes?

P: I'm not really able to see that there is anything here that can give me . . .

T: So, your thought was, in coming here, I could give you hope, sort of, maybe, or this process could . . .

P: I don't know. All I know is that when I came here it was because, I don't know.

T: Well, I think that's important to look at. It's like what you're saying is . . .

P: But see, it's like my girlfriend who works with me. We talked about this last week, and we just decided that we haven't done anything wrong in our lives. Decisions we've made or choices we've made really have not had that much of an effect on how our lives have turned out for either one of us. I think that when I came to you, maybe when you said this to me it was the right thing—I think you said my life was "just bad luck."

T: I said "bad luck"?

P: You said that I had a right to feel the way that I felt because I had a lot of bad things happen to me. It was just "bad luck."

T: I didn't say it was "bad luck." I hope I didn't say "bad luck."

P: That's the way I see it now, and there's nothing I could do to change that. I just don't feel there's anything, and I am just tired of thinking about any of this.

T: You're very frustrated.

Sarah was obviously disenchanted with her therapist. Here she expressed frustration, hopelessness, and anger at what she perceived to be an insensitive comment about her problems made early in her therapy: "Just bad luck." She apparently felt that this man was as insensitive to her needs as were other men, such as her father. She felt the need to turn to her girlfriend for support and understanding. Notice that her therapist, who characteristically was a gentle and empathic man, became defensive for a moment when he first flatly denied that he had made the remark.[3] Sarah went on to complain that her therapist did not understand the circumstances of her life and her generation that contributed to the enormous difficulty in establishing satisfying romantic relationships. Sarah got even more direct in her complaints about her therapist.

T: You seem upset with me.

P: No, it's not just with you. It's just that I keep asking you for guidelines or directions or something, and I don't ever feel like I get anything.

T: I guess if I was in your shoes, and felt that, I would be upset with me.

P: I just really . . . I just don't feel . . . I just get more confused and more frustrated. And I just think that there is nothing you can do to help me. I don't know how much I can do to help myself because . . .

T: I wonder if that reflects what happens for you with other people, and what's happening with you and me . . . that somehow people maybe try to respond to you and be there for you and you feel like there is nothing anyone can say or do.

At this point, the therapist attempted to use the primary technical strategy prescribed for brief psychodynamic psychotherapies: a transference interpretation (Levenson, 1995; Malan, 1976a; Strupp & Binder, 1984). He appeared to be using it at this point, however, to deflect Sarah's criticism by suggesting that her frustration and disappointment were part of a broader pattern of experiencing people. In the immediate interpersonal context, however, this intervention is likely to be perceived by Sarah as blaming in nature.[4]

P: No. I don't think that's right, because I think that people come to me, and I have to always reach out to them and help them.

T: But a difference is that this is a radically different situation in here. I'm not reaching out to you in any way, and your role in here is coming and saying, "Heh, I want some help with this or I want to change this." And it's a different sort of role for you to be in with someone.

P: No!

T: It's not?

P: It would be a different role to be in with you if you were really able to help me. Because I have been in this role with people trying to get support from them, but they could not give back to me, due to maybe their own personal circumstances, due to a lack of maturity on their part, to understand that they just don't quite understand or they're so caught up with there own life . . .

As illustrated in the early session of Sarah's treatment, disguised allusions to transference–countertransference enactments can often be difficult to detect. Accordingly, it is a good idea always to be alert to such clues about the status of the therapeutic relationship, even though useable clues may only occasionally appear; missing even the occasional disguised allusion to the therapeutic relationship may be too costly to the outcome of treatment, as was the case with Sarah.

Another useful tip concerning disguised allusions to transference–countertransference enactments is a mind-set that is alert to the possible parallel between the patient's topic of conversation and its implication for how the patient is experiencing the therapeutic relationship.

For example, Michelle, a young woman who had been very successful at maintaining good grades at a prestigious college, sought therapy for depression and a mild eating disorder characterized by anorexic-like food restrictions. She described the conviction that in order to be loved by those who were important to her, she needed to be "perfect": She needed to get perfect grades in school and maintain a perfect weight and body shape. During the first several therapy sessions, the main protagonist associated with the origin of her attitudes about perfection was her father, who always maintained that nothing less than the best performance was acceptable. After the fifth session, Michelle reported to her female therapist that she was no longer feeling depressed and she was doing much better at maintaining perspective on her obsession with perfect grades and physical appearance.

Although the therapist felt gratified by her patient's rapid improvement, she also had the uneasy sense that Michelle was retreating from involvement in treatment. During the sixth session, Michelle expressed concern that her recent period of good feelings might not last, because she might do something to disappoint herself, or someone else might say or do something that would deflate her good mood. Almost as an afterthought to this topic, she recalled that when she was 14, her mother had made the unexpected comment that her clothes appeared tight and that perhaps she was a little overweight and should eat less.

The implication of this memory for the immediate therapeutic relationship appears evident: Michelle had felt supported by a woman in the role of a parental-type figure. At any moment, however, this ostensibly supportive figure might say something that could undermine Michelle's current good mood; therefore, for the sake of her emotional well-being, the safest course of action was to retreat from the relationship. The allusion to the therapeutic relationship appears obvious in retrospect, but make no mistake, it takes a disciplined mind-set to consistently detect these allusions.

Managing Character Resistances

Resistance may also reflect a character style that so pervades the person's manner of coping with interpersonal relationships and the world at large that it overshadows any specific transference–countertransference pattern. For example, a person may have a distinctive style of coping with life's challenges and stresses that can be characterized along an internalizing–externalizing dimension; that is, the person either tends to accept responsibility and reflect on his or her role in situations or to look outside him- or herself for responsibility or blame and to act without much reflection. An internalizing coping style is generally well suited for the task of therapy. Taken to an extreme, however, an internalizing style can be manifested as inconsolable self-criticism. An externalizing coping style generally may require more accommodation by a therapist, but the patient's action orientation may contribute to tangible change. An extreme manifestation of this style, however, can make it extraordinarily difficult to convince the patient of taking any role at all in resolving the problems at hand. Extreme manifestations of either coping style can impede therapeutic work.

Another example of character style is that of overall level of maturity in interpersonal relating (see Chapter 3). Most of the early pioneers of brief psychoanalytic psychotherapy postulated that with relatively little time to work, engrained characterological defenses probably could not be modified and should be worked around (e.g., Malan,

1976a; Sifneos, 1972). However, contemporary clinical researchers have identified components of character style that can serve as guidelines for designing therapeutic strategies to deal with a coping style when it contributes to resistance to the therapeutic work (Beutler & Harwood, 2000; Luborsky, 1984; Piper et al., 2002).

Patients who manifest resistance in the form of a broad character style, within which a specific and relevant transference–countertransference pattern either is not detectable or is not accessible to intervention, can hold especially rigid convictions that their interpersonal reality is unalterable. Even so, a thorough inquiry that scrutinizes and deconstructs the narrative incoherence of their unquestioned views of interpersonal reality sometimes can produce emotionally arousing insights that lead to changes in thought and behavior.

Mary had been married for over 15 years and had young children. Her husband was a businessman who had worked hard to build his successful career. Mary described him, on the one hand, as trustworthy and devoted to his family, but, on the other hand, as not attuned to her feelings and needs. She reported that he was responsive when asked to be supportive but was not spontaneously sensitive. An unfortunate complement to her husband's insensitivity was Mary's strong inhibition about voicing her feelings and needs. This inability, especially when under duress, clearly was the product of traumatic childhood experiences. When Mary was a small child, her parents had divorced, and her father had disappeared precipitously. She had had no further contact with him until she was an adult. Furthermore, neither her mother nor any other relative would discuss with her the reasons for the divorce or the disappearance of her father. Everyone told her it was too upsetting. As an adult she learned that her father lived in a nearby city and eventually had remarried and raised a second family. Based on her current attitudes about discussing personal issues, it was apparent that Mary had concluded, as a child, that there was something very wrong with this activity.

Approximately 1 year before seeking psychotherapy, Mary had become involved with a man she had met through her church. They shared many intimate confidences and some physical contact. She was emotionally absorbed in this relationship and felt removed from her husband and, to a lesser extent, from her children. In the first session, she complained of feelings of guilt and that she no longer "fit" in her family. She also complained of depressive symptoms, such as sadness and anhedonia.

A character resistance was evident by the second therapy session.

Mary's strong reluctance (really, inhibition) to share personal experiences was manifested by her waiting for the therapist to ask her questions and by her talking in clipped sentences about concrete and general topics. Other than the general idea that Mary had concluded as a child that others from whom she expected emotional support would rebuff discussions of personal issues, no specific transference–countertransference pattern was detected. The idea that she might expect that her therapist also would want to avoid being exposed to her feelings and needs appeared unfathomable to Mary. She felt that, other than a vague, pervasive unhappiness, she simply had nothing specific to share, although she acknowledged a sense that even if she did have specific emotional experiences, it would be extremely difficult to reveal them.

Mary's character resistance placed a great deal of responsibility on her therapist to sustain the therapeutic inquiry. He had to work very hard; getting any meaningful communication out of Mary took enormous effort and patience. In the third session, the therapist inquired about Mary's reaction to having very little communication with her male friend. In uncharacteristically vivid terms, Mary reported that if she did not talk with him for a few days, she became increasingly sad and anxious, to the point of feeling sick to her stomach. Further inquiry revealed that these feelings were associated with the growing fear that he would never again contact her. In contradiction to this fear, however, was her emphatically stated belief that this man was very committed to their relationship and was the type of person who would talk with her about it if he were planning to end their contact.

Mary's therapist pointed out the glaring contradiction between her terror that her male friend would disappear precipitously and her conviction that he was not the type of person to do this. The therapist then proceeded to verbally construct a picture for Mary: If she did not hear from her friend for several days, she became increasingly sad and frantic. She could not, however, overtly seek support from her husband or other family members, because she was afraid of their reactions (and rightly so). Consequently, when she felt abandoned, she also felt alone and unsupported in her misery. After constructing this picture, the therapist asked Mary if it had any familiar features. In a touching show of uncharacteristic emotion, Mary cried as she admitted that the picture reminded her of her father's sudden disappearance from her life and her family's unwillingness to explain what had happened to her. She also talked about the early years of her marriage, during which she grew very resentful of her husband because she felt abandoned while he pursued his career, leaving her at home to raise their children. He had no idea how sensitive she was to feeling abandoned, and Mary was unable to share these feelings with him.

Although this dramatic insight did not significantly modify Mary's character style or the resistance encountered in her treatment, it did appear to shift her manner of coping with her feelings and needs sufficiently for her to agree to propose marital therapy to her husband. This was an idea that she had adamantly refused to consider when she began individual therapy, because the pressure to share feelings would be too great. However, she was now aware of the deep-seated influence on her of her family's pattern of disavowing the need to deal overtly with distressing experiences. Consequently, she was willing to try to face this unsettling issue, and, as she anticipated, her husband was eager to participate with her.

This shift in Mary's way of dealing with central interpersonal issues can be conceived of as the product of insight about a maladaptive interpersonal pattern gained through exploring relationships outside of therapy (in this case, recollections of childhood relationships) combined with the immediate experience of a relationship in which the other person (i.e., the therapist) appears willing to face and explore personal, uncomfortable issues.

METACOMMUNICATION

Undoubtedly there are times when the only way to deal effectively with a rupture of the therapeutic alliance—manifested by a prepotent transference–countertransference enactment—is to address it directly. Time-limited dynamic psychotherapy (Strupp & Binder, 1984) and related versions of dynamic–interpersonal therapy have prescribed a technical strategy of transference analysis that focuses on details of the immediate transactions between patient and therapist. This strategy has been considered an advance on the older psychoanalytic strategy that emphasized the T/P link (e.g., Malan, 1976a). A good example of the more contemporary here-and-now transference interpretation was illustrated in the vignette from Carl's treatment that was described in Chapter 6. In that example, the therapist observed that Carl was automatically (i.e., unconsciously) squelching his feelings in order to avoid exposing them to his therapist, even as they were discussing how Carl characteristically did this.

Even though here-and-now transference analysis, as practiced in time-limited psychotherapy, recognizes the contribution of the therapist to the enactment, the focus of examination still is directed toward the patient. Recent innovations in brief dynamic–interpersonal psychotherapy, or "relational" therapy, have gone a significant step beyond here-and-now transference analysis to include the therapist's subjective experiences, actions, and reactions as overt objects of examination. The examination of transactions in the therapeutic relationship can include, in equal measure, the participation of both patient and therapist. As noted, this inquiry strategy is called *metacommunication* (Safran & Muran, 2000).[5]

Before patient–therapist transactions can be examined, at least the outlines of some relational pattern must be detected, and the therapist must be capable of mentally stepping back from the interaction to examine it sufficiently. The generic interpersonal skills that were discussed in Chapter 1 are especially crucial to the therapist who is attempting to step back and reflect on an interaction in which he or she is currently participating.

1. The therapist must possess sufficient interpersonal pattern recognition skill to spot the influence of a specific interpersonal pattern within the ongoing patient–therapist interaction (e.g., the operation of a CMP, as described in Chapters 3 and 4).
2. The therapist must posses sufficient self-monitoring skill to be able to identify his or her covert and overt contributions to the ongoing transference–countertransference enactment.
3. In order to metacommunicate most effectively, the therapist must exercise reflection-in-action, the self-monitoring skill of recognizing and tracking the contributions of both patient and therapist to a transference–countertransference enactment while it is occurring.

Since transference–countertransference enactments that result in alliance ruptures typically have a hostile tone, successful therapeutic metacommunication also requires certain interpersonal skills directly relevant to the management of hostile interpersonal processes:

1. The capacity to tolerate a hostile interpersonal environment and maintain mental clarity and focus.
2. The capacity to maintain emotional composure, including empathy and respect for the patient, in the face of his or her overt or covert hostility.

3. The capacity to talk about problems in the therapeutic relationship with a minimum of overt or covert hostile messages (e.g., giving the interpretation "I think your disappointment with our work so far is really an expression of your disappointment with the lack of support you received from your parents" in the immediate fragile interpersonal context might be construed by the patient as a blaming message of "You have no right to act like this with me!").

An Example of Metacommunication

Katie was in therapy to deal with the chronic disturbing impact of her childhood experiences with both parents: a mother who repeatedly blamed Katie for not being sufficiently comforting to her (i.e., the mother), and a father who consistently belittled Katie as being inept at everything. Katie reliably attended all sessions with her male therapist and expressed trust and confidence in him. At the same time, she admitted that she felt that nothing much had changed in her life and that she did not feel the therapy was going anywhere. When the therapist asked Katie what she felt was missing in their relationship, she replied that she wanted her therapist to figure out what was wrong with her and what to do about it. His gut reaction to this request was resentment: He felt pressured unreasonably by the patient. He immediately thought to himself that he could not possibly answer her questions and make her feel better on the spur of the moment. It was ironic that the therapist's reflexive reaction to Katie's request was to label it as unreasonable and impossible—when the ultimate aim of any therapy is to understand the patient's problem and figure out how to solve it.

It is likely that the therapist's first reaction to Katie's request indicated something more afoot: that although what she asked of the therapist may have been reasonable on one level, it also may have carried her lifelong desire to be supported, nurtured, loved, and guided in how to get along in the world, rather than blamed and belittled for her real or imagined deficiencies. The more traditional approach to this situation would have been to offer some sort of transference interpretation, such as "What you really are seeking is for me to make up for the lack of appropriate support that you received from your parents," or "You appear to wish that I could be both omniscient in my understanding and omnipotent in my protecting of you, and you are disappointed that I am neither." An alternative approach would involve a metacommunication about the therapeutic interaction. For instance, in this case the therapist would register the paradox in his gut recoil from the patient's request, since ostensibly it appeared to be a realistic expectation of therapy. He then could share his initial reaction with his patient as well as point out its paradoxical nature. He might express puzzlement about why he had had that initial reaction, as well as puzzlement about how the patient could still be confident in the therapist's competence while feeling that no progress had been made in the treatment. The therapist's paradoxical reaction and the patient's inconsistent sentiments about the therapy and the therapist could serve as the starting points for a metacommunicative inquiry. The potential advantages of metacommunication over transference interpretations include increased effectiveness in facilitating genuine collaborative inquiry between patient and therapist and reduced likelihood of patient withdrawal in the face of perceived blame.

Therapist Self-Disclosure and Metacommunication

As the previous clinical vignette illustrates, metacommunication typically involves disclosure by the therapist of his or her subjective reactions to the patient or of observations about his or her participation in the interactions between patient and therapist. This sort of deliberate self-disclosure is distinct from the inadvertent self-disclosure associated with everything from how one decorates one's office to personal style. This latter form of self-disclosure is much more widely acknowledged by psychodynamic therapists than it used to be (Greenberg, 1995).

Traditional psychoanalytic arguments against deliberate therapist self-disclosure include the concern that such acts are usually made "reflexively" and therefore must reflect unconscious, irrational motives (Abend, 1995), or that the patient's transference experience will be contaminated by the revelation of the therapist's personal experiences (Epstein, 1995). The former argument neglects the crucial role of tacit procedural knowledge in expert therapeutic performance, whereby some acts appear reflexive when they are actually the products of rapid, complex, partially automatized decision making. Any validity that can be attributed to the latter argument is more relevant to long-term psychoanalytic therapy than to brief dynamic therapy.

The most common argument in favor of therapist self-disclosure is that it is an essential part of metacommunicating, which, in turn, is an effective strategy for engaging the patient in collaboratively examining the subtleties of the interpersonal process between patient and therapist. This endeavor serves to highlight the influence of prepotent transference–countertransference enactments and facilitates the patient's acquisition of metacognitive skills (e.g., self-monitoring) that are important interpersonal coping tools. The metacommunicating process also provides the patient with a corrective interpersonal experience; that is to say, an immediate experience in interpersonal problem solving. This argument limits deliberate therapist self-disclosure to personal reactions in the immediate patient–therapist interaction (e.g., Levenson, 1995).

As discussed in Chapter 6, some psychoanalytic therapists who espouse a relational perspective have significantly broadened the scope of self-disclosure to include any personal or professional experiences that might further a therapeutic inquiry and strengthen a therapeutic alliance. For example, Kenneth Frank (1999) has observed that experienced analytic therapists tend to rely on "self-revelation" with greater comfort and frequency than less experienced therapists. He argues that clinical experience indicates that the sharing of personal and professional anecdotes, experiences, and humor play an increasingly important role in the technique of experienced therapists.[6]

Discussions for or against deliberate therapist self-disclosure usually are based on theoretical preferences and anecdotal impressions. There is, in fact, almost no research on the impact of deliberate therapist self-disclosure. The scanty evidence available suggests that therapist self-disclosure tends to foster a productive therapeutic process, but the evidence about its impact on treatment outcome is inconclusive (Hill & Knox, 2001). There is no empirical evidence that deliberate therapist self-disclosure, conducted reasonably, is associated with negative treatment effects.

THERAPIST ERRORS IN DYNAMIC–INTERPERSONAL THERAPY

Treatment models that view transference–countertransference enactments as inevitably shaping the therapeutic relationship take the position that the most significant form of therapist error is entrapment in a patient's maladaptive interpersonal scenario (Levenson, 1995; Safran & Muran, 2000; Strupp & Binder, 1984). While considered unavoidable due to the nature of interpersonal dynamics, such errors can serve as valuable clues, if detected by the therapist, about the particular interpersonal problem that should be the focus of therapy. Other sorts of technical errors tend to be treated as relatively more

mundane, always detrimental to therapeutic progress, but easily corrected. For example, Strupp and I (1984) stated that "It is generally
expected that the therapist will become aware of errors and thus be
able to take appropriate steps to correct them" (p. 192). It is undoubtedly true, for example, that unreflective countertransference reactions
can contribute to alliance ruptures and therefore can be an important
source of resistance.

In time-limited treatment, transference–countertransference influences may sometimes reach a point of rupture as a result of deficiencies and errors in the _manner_ in which the therapist implements a
technical strategy. According to Norcross (2001), "The [therapeutic] relationship does not exist apart from what the therapist does in terms of
technique, and we cannot imagine any techniques that would not have
some relational impact. Put differently, techniques and interventions
are relational acts" (p. 349).

The emphasis of modern relational treatment models on countertransference issues and nurturing a strong alliance has led to a neglect
(or at least underestimation) of certain therapist errors that involves
what appears to be minor technical issues: (1) the therapist misunderstands the meanings of the patient's communication or intention,
(2) the therapist's communications to the patient are vague (see
Wachtel, 1993), (3) interventions are mistimed, (4) the implications of
patient communications are overlooked, and (5) transference interpretations are awkwardly used (see Henry, Schacht, et al., 1993).
Other sorts of technical errors can be more disruptive to productive
therapeutic process, such as mixed messages from the therapist that
carry implicitly hostile meanings (Henry et al., 1986) and not consistently identifying evidence in the patient's communications of a central issue (e.g., salient interpersonal theme) that should be a focus of
therapeutic work.

Relatively small and mundane technical errors may accumulate
over the course of a therapeutic relationship, resulting in small misun-
derstandings and dissatisfactions between patient and therapist that
grow into major disillusionments and emotional disengagements from
the therapeutic relationship. What I am describing is analogous to a
personal relationship, such as a marriage, that gradually withers as the
partners drift apart emotionally due to a pileup of small unresolved mis-
understandings and hurts or different aspirations that are never addressed. A patient and therapist can go through the motions for an extended period of time, like a husband and wife, while all that is left of the
relationship is a husk of what once was a lively, productive partnership.

An Example of Gradual, Mutual Disengagement from a Therapeutic Alliance

As mentioned previously, failure to track a central issue consistently is a major technical error. The therapy of Sidney, who was introduced in Chapter 4, provided illustrations of this type of error. Sidney's therapy also illustrated other relatively smaller and less noticeable errors, which could accumulate to interfere significantly with the therapeutic work. To recap: Sidney had sought therapy to deal with his discomfort over making extended commitments to anybody or anything. He felt grudgingly trapped in the obligations that he had made. His problem with commitment was associated with profoundly low self-esteem and chronic dysphoria. Sidney had undertaken several unsuccessful attempts at therapy prior to this one.

Early in the first session, Sidney described his previous strategy for selecting health care providers, including therapists.

T: Maybe the place to start is to tell me a little bit about what brings you here.

P: I didn't like my job and several other things, well, just being unhappy generally, just about everything. I decided to see a psychologist. I really didn't know any of them, but I just picked one and went to him for a while. Then I quit because I didn't think I had the time. I wasn't getting anything out of it anyway. A year or so passed. I had to get a physical. Again, I just went to some doctor. I didn't really know the doctor I went to—he was just some internal medicine doctor. He recommended that I go to another psychologist, so I started to go to the psychologist that he recommended. It was over after a few months, and again I stopped.

Although it probably is not unusual for people to seek out health care providers about whom they know nothing, Sidney made a point of reporting that the psychologists and physician with whom he consulted were just "picked" at random. One possible implication of Sidney's emphasis on this method of choosing health care providers is that he believed that one is as good, or bad, as another; in other words, his method of selection reflects his anticipation of disappointment with anyone from whom he sought help. This possibly important disguised allusion to the therapist and therapy was never acknowledged and explored by Sidney's therapist.

Later in this first session, Sidney was explaining how his parents came from modest backgrounds and had very little education. He reported that they were "intimidated" by people in their town who had more money and education. The therapist noticed that Sidney appeared more ill at ease around the subject of his parents, and he attempted to metacommunicate about this area.

T: How does it feel to talk with me about this?

P: Oh, it's embarrassing, hard.

T: How is it embarrassing?

P: It's just stuff that I've never talked to anybody about. I've always felt it, but never talked about it. I guess the only person I've talked about it with is the girl that I've gradually gotten involved with.

T: You used the word *embarrassing*. What are you imagining that I'm thinking as you're talking?

P: Probably something like "I'd get on with it if you'd quit stuttering and humming and hawing around and just say what's bothering you."

T: So, you're imagining that I might be impatient or . . .

P: Impatient, or I don't know, I guess I never really thought about what you might be thinking. It's just hard for me to (*pause*) . . . I just thought I was embarrassed. It's just, I don't want to talk about my feelings. I guess I shouldn't be embarrassed. That's what your supposed to be doing. Listening to this. But I know what I feel. It's just stuff I felt shy and embarrassed about since I was a 6 years old, and it's hard to talk about it. It's just a part of me, and I guess that's what's wrong and that's why I'm here. I've got to overcome that and it's keeping me from having any kind of life.

T: And something about the way you are isn't OK?

P: I don't think it's OK. I don't have enough courage to live. I'm always worrying about the people around me and what they think. Am I doing OK for them?

T: Can you give me an example of that?

Asking about a concrete example of an experience usually is a productive technical strategy. In this case, however, the concrete example of the patient's discomfort with what others think about him has already been identified; it is their immediate interaction, about which the therapist first attempted to metacommunicate. He started off well with this strategy, but when Sidney became even more uncomfortable and began to retreat from this line of inquiry ("I guess I never really thought about what you might be thinking."), the therapist apparently did not recognize this shift and did not comment on it. Two other potentially important implications also were overlooked. Sidney admitted that he assumed his therapist would be "impatient" with his difficulty expressing his feelings. Although the therapist did determine that Sidney's embarrassment was associated with the expectation that his therapist would be impatient with him, reasons that he might have assumed this were not explored. He also mentioned that he had felt "shy and embarrassed" since he was 6 years old, but why he identified the origin of his interpersonal discomfort as this period in his childhood was not explored.

In a session almost halfway through the therapy, Sidney was expressing frustration with his lack of progress in resolving his uncertainties about whether or not to break off his several-year relationship with his girlfriend and whether or not to leave the job that he had held for several years and in which he had received regular promotions. In both romantic and job relationships, he felt too much pressure to meet what he perceived as constant expectations and demands. The theme of grudging obligation was very strong, but the therapist did not appear to recognize it. A version of this theme, which Sidney appeared to be unconsciously attempting to enact, was to recruit the therapist into telling him what he should do about his dilemmas. The therapist's style, however, was very nondirective, so he was not easily recruited into this countertransference role. Early in the session, Sidney sounded frustrated with himself (and implicitly, with his therapist) for not communicating his feelings with sufficient clarity, and his therapist appeared confused about what Sidney was attempting to communicate.

P: . . . I never talked about things, personal stuff. . . . Listening to people at work talking to each other—they just spontaneously talk about things I have never mentioned to anyone else. I guess that's why I feel I'm just doing a bad job at this. I can't get out what I feel. I don't think I've gotten it out at all, gotten across a realistic picture of things or how I feel about them. I just don't know how to get it out. I leave here and I feel frustrated that I didn't paint the right picture. I'm just not explaining it right.

T: Is it like the picture you want to paint?

P: No, I don't think I know the picture I want to paint. I think that's a lot of the problem. It's just I've never ... I don't know myself, I guess.

T: It sounds like you're saying that as you leave here, you're not sure that I understand you to the degree that you ...

P: I'm just saying that I'm not communicating what I want to. You may be able to tell me without me having to explain the way I want to ...

T: Well, I guess one thing I'm curious about is what you hope to accomplish by painting the picture you want to paint, that's not getting accomplished. What kind of response from me or what kind of ...

P: I guess I feel like I've got to communicate my feelings better, how I really feel about working a job that I hate for all these years and seeing a girl that I'm not sure about marrying. How to explain why I've done what I've done the best way I know how. Try and explain the circumstances. Try and explain why it is. So I'll know what to do.

T: So you'll know what to do?

P: So you'll be able to understand my predicament and tell me what I need to do. You asked me last time I was here what was the purpose or what was my goal in doing this therapy. I guess, in a nutshell, it is to help me find out how to be happy or find out what I really want to do.

Halfway through the therapy, a large gap in understanding between patient and therapist became evident: They did not appear to be communicating well with each other. Unfortunately, this problem with communication and shared understanding may have been growing over several sessions. A major theme in the therapy had been Sidney's profoundly low opinion of himself, which he perceived to be a major reason for avoiding lasting commitments. He was convinced that, sooner or later, he would be exposed as embarrassingly deficient, whether in work or personal relationships. Sidney's therapist had not been able to develop any explanation for the persistence of Sidney's poor self-image in the face of an abundance of contradictory evidence. Consequently, toward the end of the session just examined, the therapist attempted simply to argue Sidney out of his poor self-image, and the therapist's exasperation was evident.

T: I guess the striking thing is that, given all that you think that is true about you, you did remarkably well for yourself. I know it doesn't feel remarkably well, but . . .

P: I'm a loser, a failure!

T: Yes, but you're not unemployed.

P: I've been unemployed a lot.

T: But you've always gotten another job.

P: Well, I never felt I succeeded.

T: Well, I understand all that, and that it feels that way. All I'm saying is that there is a kind of contrast between the way it feels and between where you see yourself and where you are, in the externals of your life. And that's not all there is, and I'm not trying to say there is. But that's a fairly remarkable contrast.

P: Well, what I feel about it is, if I'd been focused and striving toward something, what could I do then? I could do something.

T: You'd probably be president of a large corporation by now.

This last sarcastic remark reflected the therapist's growing exasperation with Sidney's inconsolable self-flagellation. It apparently had not occurred to the therapist to point out how stubbornly Sidney held on to his self-flagellation, not even pausing to consider the evidence. Whether or not this metacommunication would have been beneficial is impossible to know. The therapist's failure to attempt such a metacommunication is another small instance of accumulating technical errors. By this time, the technical errors may have become so entwined with growing emotional disengagement by the therapist, including specific countertransference reactions, that a snowballing vicious cycle was in place.

Toward the end of the therapy, evidence of a central theme of grudging obligations continued to accumulate, and Sidney's therapist continued to appear oblivious to it. Sidney reported that at work he had volunteered to take on a new project and then complained about the time required to complete it. Rather than pointing out the obvious contradiction between Sidney's volunteering to do the project and his subsequent complaints about the time required, the therapist made a sarcastic comment:

T: Just another new responsibility being dumped on you.

P: Yeah, and I don't care anything about it.

Perhaps unwittingly reacting to his therapist's sarcasm, Sidney initiated a discussion about the impending end of the treatment and their apparent failure to make much progress.

P: ... This therapy is almost over.

T: Uh-huh.

P: Do you think this has done me any good? Have you or I accomplished anything? Do you? Or should I ask that?

T: Well, you can ask it. The answer is, we would kind of have to figure it out together, I think. It's not like I have all of the information about that. A lot of it has to do with how you feel about it. What I suspect is that the goals that you came in with have not been reached.

P: I guess I feel like I haven't changed much.

T: And that was your goal. To change everything?

P: I guess the goal is so general it couldn't hardly be a goal, but it is. It's just a need to have a specific goal, I think, to really make some headway.

T: Well, I think that those goals that you have, have not been reached; to make some major changes in yourself.

P: I haven't changed anything much. It's just, what should I do differently? What am I not doing? Just nothing. Just talking about it and not doing anything to change anything. I mean, it seems like I went through one therapy with one psychologist and another therapy with another one, and I feel like I've talked about a whole lot more with you. I feel better about this than with the others, by far. But we are almost through, and I am still doing the same thing I was when I started, kind of.

T: Still going to the same job. Still seeing Susan. Living in the same house.

P: Yeah.

T: My guess is that what you have done, even though you haven't accomplished those goals, what you have done is become somewhat
more aware of exactly what those goals are. Even though you've
known them all along, you have become more aware of how powerful they are to you. It's hard to even imagine giving them up because they are so important.

The therapist was characteristically an empathic individual, to
whom people could talk easily. Sidney acknowledged this. At the same
time, it is obvious that Sidney was deeply frustrated and disappointed
with what he correctly perceived as one more failed attempt to make
significant changes in his self-image and ways of coping with his life.
He and his therapist discussed the "goals" that had not been met in
their work, but there is no evidence that they had been pursuing the
achievement of specific goals derived from a clearly defined problem
formulation. Instead, goals were discussed in vague terms, and at one
point the therapist sarcastically referred to the goal of changing "everything." The therapist's vague discussion of goals and of Sidney's
increased awareness of these goals (for which there is no evidence) is, I
believe, an unfortunately good example of a therapist who is usually
interpersonally engaged but who was merely going through the motions of talking therapeutically while progressively disengaging further from this patient.

Sidney, perhaps in desperation, asked if the therapist would give
him some last minute guidance.

P: Well, at the end of this, do you tell me what you think I ought to
do? Or do I get some kind of a report or . . .

T: Right, we give you a grade.

P: Is this the end of it, or it just depends?

A more vivid piece of evidence of the therapist's disengagement is
his particularly hostile, sarcastic response to Sidney's desperate request for something reassuring to take with him when therapy ends. In
his postsession comments, the therapist admitted that he had been
struggling to find a focus for his inquiry and that he felt "shut out" by
this patient. He failed to realize that he had been missing opportunities
to identify and inquire about several interrelated issues, including Sidney's unwillingness to consider evidence that he was not a loser and

his sense of grudging obligation to continue in relationships and at tasks at which he assumed he would fail.

In the penultimate session, the central themes of profound incompetence and entrapment in grudging obligations were particularly strong. By that time, however, the therapist appeared to have given up the attempt to identify and explore salient dysfunctional mental working models and corresponding maladaptive interpersonal patterns. He was barely going through the motions of a therapeutic inquiry, no longer looking for ways to facilitate self-reflection in Sidney or reframing of issues. He was aware that Sidney felt trapped in his job and romantic relationship, but the therapist responded as though the job and relationship were the problems rather than symptoms of more fundamental issues. Furthermore, perhaps out of continuing exasperation, the therapist finally allowed himself to be recruited into the role of advice giver, whereupon he suggested radical action.

P: I had a lot of time to sit around and think what a failure I am.

T: You mean, it's worse than you thought?

P: Yeah. What everybody said is true. I really am a loser. They're right and, plus, it's even worse than they said.

Sidney proceeded to complain vigorously about how much he "hated" his job. This complaint led to a series of interchanges between Sidney and his therapist, during which the therapist suggested that Sidney quit his job and divest himself of his other financial obligations so he would be free to do what he wanted. Sidney countered with reasons why he could not act on any of these suggestions. The therapist finally metacommunicated about these interchanges.

T: Well, you know, it's interesting that I made this suggestion, because it's kind of a radical suggestion. Quit your job, I say. And you answer very quickly—almost without giving it much thought.

The therapist finally acknowledged that he realized that Sidney was not aware of the inconsistencies and contradictions in his thinking. His attempt to metacommunicate about this, however, was relatively vague, and he did not follow up with any exploration of Sidney's unreflective responses. This was one more example of a potentially good therapeutic strategy impeded by technical errors. The therapist's postsession comments reflected his continued sense of helplessness and confusion over how to have an impact on Sidney, as well as his continued "frustration" with the way the treatment had turned out.

In the final session, Sidney blamed himself for the failure to achieve any resolution of the dilemmas he experienced in his work and in his romantic relationship with Susan. The therapist appeared to collude unwittingly in blaming Sidney for the treatment failure, and they both continued to talk vaguely about not achieving "change."

P: I failed to take advantage of opportunities. You know, I keep failing. Maybe I did talk about these things, but I just feel like I was never able to express them clearly enough. I don't know why I can't put my finger on why I feel like I haven't expressed them clearly enough, but I just still feel like I haven't or I still feel like I haven't been open enough.

T: If you were more open, what do you think would happen?

P: I'd just be, I guess I'm not brave enough to be open enough. I'd just be embarrassed talking about things that I'm not open about, and what would happen is you probably wouldn't say, "Well, that's awful," you know, but you'd say, "Well, a lot of people probably feel that way," and then I'd probably leave and feel like "I told him this and he didn't call the police." I'd probably not feel as bad about it, maybe.

T: But you seem to connect the idea of being open with the idea of being able to then change, to make change.

P: To make change?

T: To make changes. If you can really describe clearly and openly these things, maybe then you could make some changes.

The therapist summarized what he thought was the patient's point: that if he, Sidney, had been more open, he could have made more changes. Although there may be a kernel of truth to this explicit, blaming statement, the therapist appeared unaware of his own inability to clearly formulate, let alone foster the examination of, dysfunctional working mental models and corresponding maladaptive interpersonal patterns—central issues—that could have provided significant clarity as to the source of Sidney's unhappiness and immediate dilemmas.

Later in the final session, the therapist suggested that Sidney might feel that the therapist was tired of struggling to have an impact on Sidney. The evidence suggests that this was true, but the therapist never openly acknowledged it; perhaps he was not even aware of it.

P: Well, I don't guess that I assume the worst. It seems like I'm resisting change. I feel like you would think I was like thickheaded, that I'd resist change and you'd try to point out things, or ask questions to make me see a different point of view. And I just kind of resist that. That I'm stubborn to change and yet I'm sitting here saying I want change, and then I don't.

T: So maybe I'd get frustrated or tired.

P: Yeah, tired, frustrated.

T: Just tired of dealing with you, impatient.

P: No, I don't think you've been impatient. I mean, no, I don't think you've been impatient.

T: But frustrated?

P: Tired, first.

T: Tired, first—worn out.

P: Yeah.

T: Is that the way you affect people? Does Susan get tired and worn out with you? People at work, do they get worn out with you?

We know that the therapist was frustrated with Sidney, because he admitted it in his postsession notes. We also have seen evidence that he was worn out from struggling with Sidney's inconsolable self-loathing. Rather than taking this final opportunity for metacommunicating about what had transpired in their relationship, including disclosing that he was indeed frustrated and worn out, the therapist avoided this potentially uncomfortable inquiry by turning the attention to possible examples of other people who might have been worn out by Sidney's demeanor. Although looking for parallel examples of maladaptive interpersonal patterns in other relationships can be an effective technical strategy, in this context, so late in the game, there really was insufficient time to pursue the issue. Furthermore, it is likely that making these connections would have further convinced Sidney that he was a failure. Metacommunicating about what transpired in the therapeutic relationship might have afforded a better opportunity for Sidney to take something beneficial from the experience, rather than feeling like he had failed, once again.

Sidney's therapy illustrates the mutual disengagement from what might have been an effective collaborative relationship between patient and therapist. Whereas the therapist's negative feelings about, and communications with, Sidney usually would be discussed from the perspective of transference and countertransference, I have proposed that an equally important perspective is that of the cumulative, destructive impact of therapist technical errors (e.g., unclear understanding of central issues, deficiencies in communicating therapeutic interventions clearly and directly[7]). Such errors can undermine the therapeutic collaboration and perhaps heighten the transference and countertransference influences. When therapy fails, the termination often is dissatisfying for both parties. The quality of the ending of a therapy usually serves as a barometer of how the treatment fared. Termination, always considered a critical phase of therapy, is the topic of the next chapter.

NOTES

1. In contrast, in their model of brief relational therapy, Safran and Muran (2000) deal with this issue by defining their therapeutic focus as the "process" of helping the patient to develop interpersonal self-awareness skills by using whatever interpersonal pattern emerges in the therapeutic relationship. They assume that skills acquired within the therapeutic relationship will generalize to other interpersonal patterns that are causing problems outside of therapy.

2. This assumption obviously is based on clinical impressions and should be empirically tested.

3. As Henry, Schacht, and Strupp (1986) demonstrated in their analysis of the quality of interpersonal process in therapies with varying degrees of success, a little bit of hostile interaction goes a long way in therapy.

4. In their empirical analysis of events leading up to premature termination from brief psychodynamic psychotherapy, Piper et al. (1999) identified therapists' unwitting use of transference analysis as part of unproductive power struggles with their patients.

5. In their excellent manual on brief relational therapy, Safran and Muran (2000) offer an extensive, scholarly, and eloquent treatise on the therapeutic strategy of metacommunication, as well as recommendations on training therapists to do it skillfully.

6. I believe Frank (1999) is describing a shift by experienced therapists of any theoretical persuasion toward a more mentoring approach, which relies on the wisdom acquired by many therapists through personal and professional experiences associated with lifelong learning.

7. Paul Wachtel (1993) has written an important book on lucid communication in therapy.

8

Termination

with Karishma K. Patel

THE CHANGING NATURE OF TERMINATION

Termination commonly denotes a final ending. This meaning is reflected in the typical approach to ending treatment in psychoanalysis and long-term psychoanalytic therapy. This approach of termination as a final ending was predicated on the assumption that successful treatment would resolve the patient's core problems (Ticho, 1972). Furthermore, the treatment models of the early brief psychoanalytic therapists espoused this view of termination more or less explicitly and more or less rigidly. They all sought to resolve circumscribed "core" conflicts, the resolution of which was presumed to prepare the patient to carry on life successfully for an indeterminate period of time. Accordingly, none of the pioneers in early brief psychoanalytic therapy discussed repeated courses of therapy as a routine option. Instead, their opinions ranged from rigidly observed terminations (Mann, 1973; Mann & Goldman, 1982) to more flexible approaches (Davanloo, 1980; Malan, 1976a; Sifneos, 1979).

Karishma K. Patel, MA, is currently a doctoral student in Clinical Psychology at the Georgia School of Professional Psychology of Argosy University, Atlanta, where she received her MA in Clinical Psychology. She received her BA in Psychology from the University of Virginia, Charlottesville.

A less commonly known meaning of *termination* is to limit or bound, to circumscribe the allocation of something, such as time. In their approach to ending treatment, contemporary brief therapists tend to use this meaning of termination. The amount of time allocated for a course of therapy is circumscribed, but termination does not necessarily refer to a final ending of the therapy relationship. There is an implicit or explicit (now more common) agreement that the patient can return for subsequent courses of therapy, if and when the need arises. Indeed, many modern brief therapists view repeated courses of treatment over the course of an adult's life as routine, comparable to the routine visits to medical practitioners for various ailments. Just as living continuously exposes us to various organic pathogens and injuries, it also exposes us to various psychological stresses. In addition, by circumscribing the problem areas addressed, brief therapy may neglect some active or potential problems. Such problems may be addressed in a future course of treatment.

There is no consensus on arrangements for terminating brief therapy, a situation that is comparable to the lack of consensus on how to terminate psychoanalysis (Firestein, 2001). The most common strategies are (1) setting a specific number of sessions, (2) setting a specific calendar date, or (3) informing the patient that the treatment will not go longer than a few weeks or months without specifying a date (Davanloo, 1980; Malan, 1976a; Mann, 1973; Sifneos, 1979). I have found nothing in the empirical evidence thus far that favors a single approach to setting a definite date or number of sessions. I believe that it makes most sense to discuss the anticipated length of, or specific end of, treatment after a therapeutic focus has been introduced. At this point, the patient has a circumscribed issue and corresponding goals that should appear more attainable within a limited period of time (Strupp & Binder, 1984). There is some consensus around the view that the patient should be reminded periodically of the limits on time, in order to discuss reactions to the prospect of termination and to prepare for it (Luborsky, 1984; Stadter, 1996; Safran & Muran, 2000).

Two strategies that have had some use in open-ended and brief therapies are (1) tapering the frequency of sessions toward the end of treatment, and (2) conducting follow-up sessions several weeks or months after regularly scheduled sessions have ended. These strategies are much more commonly used now because they provide several benefits: (1) continued nurturance for patients who need time to relinquish the safety, comfort, and security of the therapy relationship and cope more successfully with the ending of therapy; (2) a way of monitoring progress in patients' ability to work through issues outside of therapy and to use newly acquired or enhanced interpersonal skills; and (3) additional time for examination of how significant life events and stresses are handled (Stadter, 1996, Strupp & Binder, 1984).

There appears to be a growing appreciation for the wide variety of ways in which patients construe termination and react to it. For instance, the long-held notion that termination is one of the most crucial challenges for patient and therapist may characterize some therapies but not all. It may be the case that the combination of brevity and the diminished psychological significance of the doctor–patient relationship (discussed in Chapter 6) not only lessens the impact of transference but also lessens the impact of termination as well. On the other hand, termination may be especially difficult with patients for whom separation and loss are psychologically significant issues, with whom there is the potential for a hostile–dependent attachment to the therapist. However, even in these cases, it is not inevitable for termination to evoke painful memories of earlier losses or separations and to revive feelings associated with past traumas. Furthermore, patients who do not have significant feelings about termination may not necessarily be denying or defending against intimacy and dependence, as some authors have suggested (Stadter, 1996).

A crucial variable to consider when prognosticating a patient's reaction to termination is the quality of his or her interpersonal support network. Patients who have meaningful and gratifying relationships are less prone to experience termination as rejection or abandonment. Conversely, patients without such a support network are more prone to cling to the therapeutic relationship as a crucial attachment and experience termination as rejection or abandonment. If termination is psychologically significant to a patient, how the loss is experienced and defensively reacted to will be influenced by the central issues that were the focus of therapy (Malan, 1976a; Mann, 1973; Strupp & Binder, 1984).

We propose that given the strong and growing inclination for both patients and therapists to view psychotherapy from a "primary care" perspective—that is, as a health care resource that can be accessed repeatedly—conceiving of termination as an inevitable potential crisis may be overestimating its significance. Budman and Gurman (1988) argued that excessive focus on termination with every patient may be unwarranted and have little relevance for some. As another brief therapist, who has systematically studied terminations in brief therapy, put it, "[The therapist should] . . . neither overemphasize nor underemphasize the meaning of the end of therapy" (Quintana, 1993, p. 430). Therapists should evaluate each therapeutic relationship on its own merits and strive to distinguish between legitimate, appropriate reactions to termination and unhealthy, excessive ones.

THE IMPACT OF CONTEXTUAL FACTORS ON TERMINATION

Changes in the socioeconomic climate have led to changes in both the therapeutic process, as a whole, and in the termination phase of therapy, in particular. Wachtel (2002) argues that the termination of the therapeutic work should not denote the end of therapy. In fact, although the therapist–client dyad may have concluded its circumscribed work, the individual has not necessarily gone as far as he or she can go in terms of psychological development. Wachtel's contention that the patient can carry on his or her therapy after the formal therapeutic relationship has ended is especially significant in view of the temporal constraints that managed care places on therapy. In a sense, managed care forces an individual to continue his or her psychological development without the aid of a therapist. Conversely, a consequence of this temporal constraint is the risk of creating iatrogenic splitting. Even when the managed care company puts financial limits on therapy, it is the therapist who ultimately decides that he or she is unwilling, for economic reasons, to continue the treatment after reimbursement has stopped. However, the therapist may blame the managed care company as the culprit, rather than openly acknowledging his or her choice not to work for free. If patients need to express sentiments about having their treatment limited, it is healthier for them to express themselves to a therapist who can accept their complaints, than to direct futile protestations toward an impersonal and anonymous insurance company.

Time constraints, exclusive of current socioeconomic barriers, may also prevent a continuing relationship. For example, trainees must leave at the end of a designated period. Thus, individuals in training who are required to terminate treatments because they are leaving their training sites may have a separate and specific set of difficulties and concerns. Trainees are likely to face a more difficult ending than practicing therapists, because usually they do not have the flexibility to taper the frequency of sessions gradually, to conduct follow-up sessions, or to offer patients a future renewal of their relationship. Furthermore, trainees who have not yet dealt with their own countertransference feelings toward separation and loss may have an even more difficult experience with termination. Therefore, careful and empathic supervision during the termination phase may be particularly important for trainees. Malan (1976a) suggested that as part of their learning experience, trainees work within a longer framework, but no more than 30 sessions. In the absence of relevant research, however, we do not have a clear picture of the particular hazards faced by trainees and their patients during termination.

DISCUSSION OF TERMINATION ISSUES AND SUCCESS OF THERAPY

Along with the traditional assumption that termination is inevitably an emotionally crucial event for patients is the corollary assumption that failure to properly work through the termination phase will compromise much of the previous therapeutic work and serve as an impediment in patients' ability to achieve their goals (Hoyt, 1979; Levenson, 1995). If the more contemporary view is taken—that patients vary enormously in the significance that termination holds for them—the question remains: How much should termination be discussed in order to increase the likelihood of a positive treatment outcome? There appears to be a general consensus that if termination is going to be a significant psychological issue for the patient, it should be thoroughly discussed (Quintana, 1993; Safran & Muran, 2000; Strupp & Binder, 1984).

However, there is almost no empirical evidence to guide therapists in dealing with termination. In one small attempt to gain some empirical data on which aspects of termination can impact the success of therapy and how the termination phase should be handled, Quintana and Holahan (1992) studied counselors' self-reported procedures during the termination phase. They found that in short-term counseling, unsuccessful cases were characterized by less review of the course of counseling and more limited discussion of the clients' feelings about ending counseling. The researchers hypothesized that these findings may have been a product of both the counselors' and the clients' hesitance to discuss the negative aspects of therapy, which would have been more prevalent in unsuccessful cases. Marx and Gelso (1987), using client self-reports, found that a greater amount of termination work occurred when the treatment was of longer duration and the patient had established a close relationship with the therapist. In sum, the limited empirical evidence suggests that it is especially important to explore a patient's feelings about termination when the treatment has not gone well and when the patient shows signs of having formed a significant attachment to the therapist.

TIME-LIMITED THERAPY AND ACCELERATED CHANGE

A fundamental assumption of all brief therapies is that limiting the amount of available time serves as an incentive for patient and therapist to work as diligently as possible. Applebaum (1975) proposed that this phenomenon represented a variation of "Parkinson's law," which states that the amount of time required to achieve a specific goal expands or contracts as a function of the time available or allocated. Until recently, however, there has been no empirical test of this proposition.

As discussed in Chapter 1, two recent studies have provided qualified and limited support for the relevance of Parkinson's law to psychotherapy. In the first study, Reynolds and colleagues (1996) compared the amount of change in 8-session versus 16-session cognitive-behavioral and dynamic–interpersonal therapies. On a variety of measures, they found that the rate of change was significantly greater in the 8-session compared to the 16-session therapies. The researchers concluded that this finding reflected the patients' efforts to accelerate therapeutic understanding in order to make the most efficient use of limited time. It appeared that more limited time served as an incentive for patients to "get down to business."

The other study, performed by Barkham and colleagues (1996) replicated the results of the Reynolds et al. study (1996). Using similar methodology, the researchers found that a significantly higher proportion of participants showed reliable change at the end of the eighth session of the 8-session treatment than at the end of the eighth session of the 16-session treatment. A larger proportion of participants, however, achieved clinically significant change by the end of the 16-session treatment in comparison to the 8-session treatment. The researchers also found that symptoms associated with acute distress showed the fastest change, whereas vegetative symptoms and characterological and interpersonal issues demonstrated slower change. The Barkham et al. (1996) findings suggest that acute symptoms are most responsive to constraints on the duration of treatment. This observation is supported by the dose–effect studies that indicate that acute symptoms respond most rapidly to therapeutic intervention, followed by interpersonal functioning and characterological change (Howard et al., 1986; Kopta et al., 1994).

On the basis of these studies, the following tentative conclusions can be made:

1. Limiting the duration of therapy may influence the rate of change rather than the amount of change.
2. The breadth of change is greater for longer therapy; in other words, more time leads to more change.
3. Acute symptoms exhibit more rapid change than character-ological problems.

An important caveat to interpreting the results of these treatment comparison studies must be acknowledged. The Reynolds et al. (1996) and the Barkham et al. (1996) studies are limited by low external validity, since they were conducted with artificially shortened therapies under highly controlled conditions.

STRATEGIES AND GUIDELINES FOR TERMINATION

In contrast to a rigid adherence to the notion of termination as a final ending, our guidelines reflect the increasing heterogeneity of views regarding the meaning and role of termination, as well as the increasing flexibility with which termination is approached. It remains wise, when ending treatment, to pay particular attention to patients who have dependent tendencies and/or issues with separation and loss. For most patients in brief therapy, however, these issues may be irrelevant, and excessive focus on them may interfere with a smooth, natural, and positive end to treatment (Budman & Gurman, 1988). The method of gradually tapering off sessions, offering follow-up sessions, and extending an explicit invitation to return to therapy if the patient encounters future problems is not likely to interfere with the consolidation of therapeutic gains—and, in fact, is more likely to contribute to it.

As proposed above, patients are better able to cope with the end of the therapeutic relationship if they have meaningful relationships outside of therapy. Consequently, this area of the patient's life should be addressed throughout therapy and should be a particular area of interest as therapy draws to a close.

I do not have a set opinion about the advisability of setting a specific end to therapy by number of sessions or a calendar date. However, I do strongly advise therapists to explain, clearly and explicitly, to patients that they will be working as efficiently as possible and that the treatment will be of limited duration. I also recommend that if a termination date is set early in treatment, the therapist does so only after the patient's psychological resources and interpersonal support network have been evaluated and a focus for the therapeutic work has been formulated and accepted by the patient (Garfield, 1998; Strupp & Binder, 1984). The amount of time initially allocated for therapy is influenced by the therapist's estimate of the patient's psychological resources. Obviously more time is allocated when less psychological resources are evident and/or less outside interpersonal support is available; unfortunately, these two circumstances tend to go together. In any event, the patient is more likely to accept a time limit as reasonable after he or she has agreed to the therapist's proposed problematic issue, toward which to focus the therapeutic work.

AREAS FOR FUTURE RESEARCH

Due to the low external validity of the studies on accelerated change, further research should explore how time limits affect the rate of change in natural treatment settings. Furthermore, since the meaning of *time* and *termination* is influenced by the cultural and subcultural views of patients, ethnic/racial, cultural, and socioeconomic factors may have a significant impact on the meanings attributed to setting time limits on therapy and to termination. These variables should be the subject of future research on time limits and termination. For example, allocating 3 months for therapy may seem like an eternity for one person, signifying serious mental illness and therapist pessimism, whereas for another individual this same period of time may seem insufficient to accomplish even circumscribed goals.

AN EXAMPLE OF DEALING WITH TERMINATION

When ending the therapy relationship is not psychologically significant for the patient or therapist, their final interactions are a natural conclusion to the work that they have been doing up to that time. Whether patient or therapist raises the issue of terminating, it is good practice for the therapist to inquire directly about the patient's feelings in that regard as well as his or her expectations and concerns about the future without therapy. Patients often do not have much to say on these topics; they typically express appreciation for what has been accomplished and sometimes some sadness about ending what has been a gratifying and beneficial relationship. As mentioned above, when the work has not gone so well, the therapist should make a point of encouraging candid discussion about how both parties may have contributed to the disappointing outcome.

When ending the therapy relationship is psychologically significant for the patient, it is good practice for the therapist to explore how the central issues that have been the focus of the therapeutic work influence how the patient construes the ending of their relationship, as well as how the patient's characteristic self-protective (i.e., defensive) maneuvers influence his or her reactions to terminating. Skillful and empathic therapeutic efforts during this time can consolidate gains made during the preceding work on central therapeutic issues. On the other hand, ignoring or overlooking opportunities for such work can detract from previous therapeutic gains, because patient and therapist may unwittingly reenact—and thereby reinforce—maladaptive mental working models and corresponding interpersonal patterns, just as treatment ends.

Below is an example of a patient who was very emotionally attached to her male therapist and who had a difficult time giving up this relationship. She was prone to experience termination as another instance of the rejection that she had come to expect from significant relationships, and she reacted in her characteristically defensive way. This was the penultimate session of a planned time-limited treatment that lasted approximately 30 sessions.

Emma was in her mid-30s, had been married for over a decade, and had two school-age children. The central issue of her treatment was formulated in CMP terms as follows: She wished to be accepted, valued, and loved by her significant others, particularly her husband and children. She expected, however, that others would value her only if she made herself "indispensable" in caring for their wants and needs, and if she did not burden them with her wants and needs. She was a diligent caretaker for her family and insisted that they not concern themselves with her needs. For example, she would downplay the importance of her birthday and encourage her family to ignore it. Her husband and children, as well as other people who knew her, responded to such behavior by going along with what she appeared to want. They treated her as if she had no wants or needs. Emma appeared to approve of this treatment but secretly felt hurt and resentful that those to whom she felt closest would ignore her needs so blatantly. These experiences reinforced (1) her expectation that significant others did not want to be burdened with her wants and needs, and (2) her self-image as unlovable and only of value when taking care of others. Emma sought therapy because she suffered from chronic feelings of unhappiness and anxious insecurity and because she was afraid that her husband no longer loved her.

A thumbnail sketch of her childhood relationships with parents provided clues to Emma's current dysfunctional mental working model and interpersonal patterns. She reported that her father was a stern, unaffectionate man whose primary contact with his children was to discipline them, often cruelly. She reported that her mother worked hard as a homemaker and let everyone know how hard she worked. She typically made Emma feel as if her presence were a bother and a burden. Emma would often flee to a relative's house, who lived nearby, in search of attention and nurturance. The penultimate sessions began like this:

T: How are you doing?

P: OK. (*Laughs nervously.*)

T: What?

P: No, I was just thinking that this is number 29, right?

T: Yes.

P: Whatever.

T: Well, what are your thoughts about that?

P: Well, it makes my heart jump a beat (*laughs nervously*), but I think it is OK.

T: How come?

P: How come? (*Laughs nervously.*)

T: How come it's OK? What's OK about it?

Emma began the session by raising the issue of their planned termination after the next session. She evidently was apprehensive about it, but immediately attempted to reassure the therapist that he should not be concerned (about her feelings?). He appeared to recognize this characteristic maneuver of downplaying her feelings and questioned what she meant. With minimal encouragement from her therapist, Emma was able to say that the therapy relationship had been important to her. In addition, she was able, if somewhat meekly, to utter a small complaint about not being able to continue with her therapist. Perhaps this was a small sign of the progress that she had made in therapy around acknowledging her wants.

T: Well, tell me what you're thinking now?

P: Well, it's not like I can't live without you or the counseling.

T: Hmm.

P: But it does help, and I'm not totally dependent on you. I go through 2 weeks and do OK. I don't usually call you between sessions. I know I can, you know, live a pretty normal life on my own without you. But also if it helps, then I think I should, you know, if it's OK with you, then I should be able to see you. I mean, it's not like I'm not able to separate myself totally from you. I don't think there is a problem, you know what I mean? I don't feel like there's a problem with counseling, with you, that I can't stay away from you.

To paraphrase Shakespeare, the lady "doth protest too much." Emma was clearly very attached to her therapist, did not want to end their relationship, but at the same time did not want to appear needy and demanding to him—a judgment she apparently expected from him in reaction to her feelings and wants.

Emma shared with her therapist the feelings of acceptance and understanding that she had felt in their interactions. She contrasted these good experiences with the judgmental and critical sentiments that she had experienced from a male counselor whom she had seen only once. Emma's therapist wondered about the implications of this complimentary comparison in the context of their current discussion of termination. He finally began to intimate that a man with whom she had no relationship could reject her, but how could he end their relationship after it had been so extended and beneficial. The therapist was not able to express his entire thought, because Emma appeared to grasp the implications immediately. She began to laugh nervously and admitted that it kept her from crying.

T: You're sad about it.

P: (wiping away her tears and pausing) It's OK.

T: It's "OK." What does "It's OK" mean? What's OK?

P: That I'm not upset that we're stopping.

T: How are you feeling toward me about this stopping?

P: I'm not mad at you. It's not that at all, no. I'm not mad. I just feel, I don't know, it's like I'm used to coming here and seeing you . . .

T: Hmm.

P: And I'll miss that. It's not so much that, I mean, like I said, I know that if I need to talk to you, I can. It's just that I knew each week that I would be coming here, every 2 weeks or 3 weeks, I would be coming here. It was established, something that happened.

T: And it means a lot?

P: Hmm.

T: Well, when we talk about it, and you feel the strong feelings that you felt a minute ago, and then you clamp down real tight on those, and then you say as soon as you can, "It's OK." So what are you telling me there? I mean, what are you . . .

P: Well, I'm telling you I don't want to get upset about it, because I'm afraid that you'll think "We've got a problem now," you know, "She can't cut it, she can't let go."

T: So you have to act as though this hurts less than it hurts?

P: Yeah, yeah, I think maybe it would make it easier.

T: On whom?

P: For you. If I just go on like [nothing is changing].

T: Why do you have to make it easier for me? Now think about that.

P: Because I was taught to do that (*laughs nervously*).

T: Can you tell me more about that. What do you mean?

P: Well, it just seems like the thing to do, to not cling, to not get emotional about it. It's pretty inconvenient to get emotional about it.

In these interchanges, Emma played out some of the main components of the central issue that they had worked on as the focus of treatment. She wanted to continue the therapeutic relationship but expected that the therapist would be judgmental and critical of these wants, so she tried to squelch her feelings and reassure the therapist that he had nothing to be concerned about, she would not make a fuss about ending. The therapist appeared to be aware of this characteristic defensive process and addressed it by encouraging Emma to talk further about her immediate feelings. At the same time, he explicitly acknowledged her reluctance to explore her reactions to ending their relationship. Emma admitted that she had never been able to talk candidly with a man until this experience and therefore felt very close to her therapist. She would miss their relationship but assumed that, although her therapist believed that they had worked well together, he would not miss her: "I'm just another patient of yours. . . ." At this point the therapist explicitly raised the issue of rejection.

T: Is there a part of you that still feels some rejection regardless of what you are trying to think?

P: Probably.

T: Probably. Well, can you give a little more voice to what that part is experiencing?

P: Hmm. (*long pause*) I don't know that I can. It's normal for me, it just comes as easy as breathing for me to think *rejection*. So that did come up, the thought did go through my mind that, you know, that "He's rejecting me"—that did go through my mind. But I didn't dwell on it enough to say "Yeah," because I really haven't allowed myself to think about "He's rejecting me." I start thinking, "That's not the way it is, this is what it's all about, and this is what happened, and it did happen and it was good, and it's not about any of that."

T: Does that provide some comfort to think that way?

P: Yes. It feels healthy. I don't think it's any reflection on me, as far as the way I feel about myself, that we're stopping these sessions. I don't think there's any bad reflection on me for stopping these sessions. I don't feel bad about myself, because we're stopping these sessions.

In response to her therapist's invitation to discuss her proneness to experience the termination as a rejection, Emma described a struggle between interpreting termination as rejection and a new experience of interpreting it as an inevitable occurrence that does not reflect upon her. She viewed this alternative perspective as "healthy." Her therapist continued to comment on her reluctance to share her feelings about ending, and she admitted to feeling sad about ending and that it was analogous to losing a valued relationship through the death of the other person. She experienced her therapist as "slipping away" from her. At the same time, she experienced termination as an event in which she played an active role, more so than in previous endings, when she simply had felt rejected for being unworthy.

P: I guess the difference is that I am feeling that I'm letting you go. I'm not used to doing that.

T: You're more used to trying to cling?

P: Yeah.

T: Like, to you're mom?

P: In a way.

T: So in some ways what you're talking about is feeling sad, but it may reflect more of a strength or an attempt to be stronger?

P: I think so.

T: Or . . .

P: I think so, I think that's what I am telling myself. This is not like the other times that someone has walked away and I had to stop something that I thought was good.

T: Do you think it's a good idea to stop?

P: To stop the sessions? No! (*Laughs.*)

T: (*Laughs.*) OK.

P: It was good to laugh.

T: It's hard to stop, isn't it?

The therapist offered Emma a crystal-clear invitation to express her feelings about termination, and she bluntly expressed her dislike of it. Her experience of the therapist accepting this defiance allowed her, perhaps for the first time, to make a hostile (i.e., sarcastic) comment about the therapist getting what he wanted out of their work (a success) and therefore ready to end their collaboration, regardless of what she wanted. She then returned to her sadness about ending. But she was noticeably more subdued, and her therapist responded by directly commenting on her characteristic tendency to squelch her wants in order to take care of significant others. Emma admitted that she was not sure if she would let her therapist know is she was very upset about ending their relationship, because those feelings are so "personal." She also admitted that she did not believe the ending was emotionally significant to her therapist.

P: Well, I look at it kind of like a physician would if a patient had an illness. They have other patients (*laughs nervously*) with the same illness. They feel bad, but it's not their problem.

Emma's therapist realized that even if she were able to experience the coming termination as something other than a personal rejection, she still would be prone to view the ending of the therapy relationship as something that emotionally impacted her but not him. In their interchange, Emma had been able to go beyond her characteristic interpersonal pattern of stifling her own wants in order to avoid anticipated rejection, but she still could not imagine that she was worthwhile enough for her therapist to miss her after the relationship ended. Consequently, to counter Emma's entrenched self-devaluation, the therapist decided that he would have to disclose some of his own feelings about the end of their relationship.

T: What if you are not just a statistic, and that my knowledge of how difficult this is for you hurts me too, in some ways. Would there be any way that you could know that? Does that seem possible?

Even though the therapist had increased the flexibility of his approach when he began conducting brief treatments, originally he had been trained to use a relatively conservative psychodynamic stance that essentially prohibited therapist self-disclosure. His ambivalence was evident in the roundabout manner in which he initially suggested that he would miss working with Emma. Nevertheless, he believed that for Emma to overcome her entrenched dysfunctional mental model of significant relationships, his disclosure of feelings was beneficial—perhaps even necessary. He also reframed the meaning of his adherence to the termination schedule. He encouraged Emma to consider an alternative to her presumption that it would be easy for him to end their relationship, because she did not mean much to him; the alternative was that he was ready to follow through on the planned ending, even though he would miss their working together, because he thought it would be in her best interests.

T: Well, does that make it worse to think about the possibility that it does matter to me and that, uh . . .

P: No, it doesn't make it worse. I think it makes me feel . . . if you feel bad about it, if you really feel bad about it (*giggles*), it makes me feel—oh, gosh—it makes me feel better. I don't know why.

T: Well, it makes you feel like more than a number or statistic.

P: And it makes me feel that it wasn't my imagination that we had good rapport, and that what went on was productive and helpful for both sides, rather than, you know, just trying to be nice because, I mean, you come across to me as a real nice person.

Emma indicated that she was beginning to appreciate, genuinely, that the coming ending would be painful, if in different degrees, to both herself and her therapist. She experienced him as caring enough about her to be affected by their parting. Although she remained sad and apprehensive, she also evidenced some satisfaction in feeling valued. Initially Emma had experienced the approaching termination as another variation on the theme of being devalued and rejected. Now, however, she had reframed its meaning in a new and healthy way. In other words, her therapist's skillful work around the termination facilitated a corrective emotional–interpersonal experience for Emma. Her therapist reinforced this experience with a final bit of self-disclosure, even though his prior conservative training made it difficult to be completely open: He could acknowledge that he would miss their work together, but he could not bring himself to say that he would miss Emma, personally.

T: . . . this is hard to do, and you know I've enjoyed this [work together]. I'm going to miss this, and it's been meaningful to both of us, but we still have to say good-bye.

The end of this therapy also brings us to the end of our discussion of how brief dynamic–interpersonal therapy is conducted. The final topic, covered in Chapter 9, concerns how students are trained to conduct therapy.

9

Training

This chapter is written primarily for psychotherapy teachers and researchers interested in therapy training. Practicing therapists also may be interested in my thoughts about current deficiencies in training, as well as my recommendations for improvements. This discussion may stimulate ideas about how practicing therapists can enhance their own continuing education. My recommendations for improving therapy training were inspired, in part, by the same source that guided my thinking about the foundation of therapist competencies: research in the cognitive sciences on the nature of skillful complex performance and how it is achieved. My primary inspiration, however, came from instructional psychology research on how to enhance generic learning, both knowledge acquisition and skill development. Innovative teaching formats that incorporate state-of-the-art technologies have been introduced and evaluated in K–12 educational systems, military training, business, and law and medicine. Even though psychologists have been instrumental in developing these innovative teaching methods, graduate training programs in clinical psychology as well as other therapy training programs have not taken advantage of them. Most of the recommendations for improving therapy training offered in this chapter have not been enacted. They are intended to serve as guidance for therapy training research and development projects. I personally am embarking on such an endeavor and invite other psychotherapy teachers to join me in this sort of work.

WHAT DO WE KNOW ABOUT PSYCHOTHERAPY TRAINING?

What do we know about psychotherapy training? My answer, in a few words, is that we have many opinions but little research-informed knowledge. I believe that it is safe to say that the faculty of most accredited clinical training programs assume, at least implicitly, that their training programs are effective at producing competent entry-level therapists. Only on rare occasions can allusions to problems in therapy training can be found in the clinical literature. For example, many years ago the renowned psychoanalytic teacher Karl Menninger mentioned his own "bewilderment" as a novice taught theoretical concepts and explanations that nevertheless left him unsure of what was happening in his work with patients and what to do about it (Menninger & Holzman, 1973). Prior to Menninger's admission, another notable psychoanalytic theorist and teacher, Otto Fenichel, had observed that "it is difficult [for novice therapists] to recognize again the well understood theoretical concepts in what they see and experience in the patient, and still more in what they themselves say and do during the analytic hour" (Fenichel, 1941, p. 2).

These observations imply a problem in the transfer of knowledge from course work and supervision to performance with actual patients. More recently, the esteemed interpersonal psychoanalyst Edgar Levenson (1998), struggled with trying to understand this problem without having an adequate language of pedagogy to help him; all he had was his familiar clinical language. Nevertheless, he understood that learning a new skill usually involves a period of disorienting self-consciousness. To make his point by analogy, he related the cautionary tale of the centipede who tripped over "his" own feet when he began to think about how he managed to walk.

These learned clinical teachers were referring to what contemporary cognitive scientists call *inert* knowledge: that is, conceptual knowledge that is not readily useable to guide practical understanding and skillful performance in the real world. I have come to the conclusion that the problem of inert knowledge is a major impediment to effective psychotherapy training. Before exploring this topic of inert knowledge, I present a representative sampling of what we know about psychotherapy training. Because I view therapy from a dynamic–interpersonal perspective, my discussion emphasizes psychodynamic training. I believe, however, that my observations have broader applicability.

Psychotherapy texts and manuals seem like an obvious place to look for discussions about training. In fact, they usually contain relatively little discussion about how novices are trained to conduct treatment. The matter of training seems to be almost an afterthought. This state of affairs may stem from the prevailing viewpoint that effective psychotherapy results from implementing techniques that either are supported by the findings of a preferred research paradigm or are prescribed by a preferred theory.

Whether supported by empirical findings or by a preferred theory, the focus on prescribed techniques rather than on the nature of skillful therapeutic performance contributes to minimizing the role of training. In fact, relatively little is known about therapy *training* processes and outcomes compared to what is known about therapy processes and outcomes. Over the years, there has been minimal effort directed toward investigating training effectiveness (Binder, 1993). In the past few years this low level of research activity has shrunk noticeably lower (Beutler, 1997). Reviews of psychotherapy training invariably conclude with calls for more research. These incantations, however, have not produced the desired result. The last two editions of the encyclopedic *Handbook of Psychotherapy and Behavior Change* (Bergin & Garfield, 1994; Lambert, 2004), the principle repository of therapy research findings, have omitted a chapter on training. The editors state that topics in each edition reflect "current trends," implying that psychotherapy researchers are not particularly interested in the topic of psychotherapy training.

WHAT DO WE KNOW ABOUT FORMAL GRADUATE TRAINING IN PSYCHOTHERAPY?

It is not an exaggeration to say that the effectiveness of formal graduate psychotherapy training—whether in psychology or psychiatry—is assumed largely on faith. The assumption that these programs provide effective therapy training and therefore produce competent therapists, however, has no body of substantiating empirical evidence. As Len Bickman, the knowledgeable social scientist, so bluntly stated, this assumption must be considered a "myth"—that is, a belief reflecting uncritical support for existing or traditional practices (Bickman, 1999; Christensen & Jacobson, 1994; Kazdin, 2000).

The format most widely used for psychotherapy training in graduate clinical training programs consists of course work, followed by supervision of actual cases through practica and internships. Many programs—especially those favoring a psychodynamic orientation—

encourage students to obtain personal therapy, in order to refine emotional sensitivities and interpersonal skills.

Repeated surveys indicate that practicing therapists consider personal therapy to be a crucial part of their training (Macran & Shapiro, 1998). Therapists tend to believe that a personal therapy, particularly early in their careers, is beneficial for several reasons, the primary ones being that it provides firsthand experience of how therapy works and validates its benefits (Fridrum, Coyle, & Lyons, 1999). Whereas there is no scarcity of opinions about the value of a therapist's personal therapy, the sparse empirical evidence that exists provides no substantial support for the idea that personal therapy contributes to the training of a competent and effective therapist (Macran & Shapiro, 1998).

Not an argument for omitting it

Evidence from the admittedly meager research available on clinical training programs suggests that the most effective components are a combination of structured didactic and experiential activities that are designed to teach specific procedures and skills in a progression from simple to more complex performances (Beutler, 1997; Binder, 1993). Over the past four decades, various innovative structured teaching methods have been incorporated into some clinical training programs. An early development involved several versions of "microskills" training, in which discrete teaching modules were developed to teach basic components associated with clinical interviewing (e.g., "active listening," asking open-ended questions; Ivey, 1971). It appears, however, that although these microcomponents of interviewing can be taught effectively, the components do not easily gel into the more complex performance skills actually used in clinical interviewing (Binder, 1993; Lehman & Ericsson, 1997). The use of videotaped recordings of real or simulated therapy sessions has allowed for the relatively structured study of various sorts of patient–therapist interactions as well as specific technical interventions. However, there has been no investigation of whether such discrete structured teaching methods, nested within traditional training programs, significantly enhance clinical performance during or after training (Binder, 1993).

In general, recent advances in the teaching of psychodynamic forms of therapy have been limited to technical innovations, such as the use of tape recordings to illustrate treatment activities and review trainees actually doing therapy, as well as the use of treatment manuals to provide more precise specification of therapeutic principles and procedures. These improvements, however, have not been organized and grounded in a pedagogical theory that would guide instruction in therapy knowledge and skills, leading to effective complex performances. There really is no explicit pedagogical theory that guides the way course work is organized for teaching psychotherapy. In general, teaching formats are organized around curricula that expose students to theories and procedures associated with one or more treatment models, followed by an abrupt transition to "practicing" with real patients. Furthermore, there is a set of tacit basic assumptions associated with psychotherapy training that a doctoral degree and a faculty position qualify an individual to teach therapy courses, and that a doctoral degree and clinical experience qualify another individual to offer therapy supervision. These are more myths; in graduate school novice therapists receive little or no training in how to teach or supervise therapy.

WHAT DO WE KNOW ABOUT THE IMPACT OF TREATMENT MANUALS ON PSYCHOTHERAPY TRAINING?

Two decades ago it was assumed that the advent of treatment manuals would "revolutionize" psychotherapy research and spur (secondarily) great advances in psychotherapy training. Treatment manuals have manifested significant progress in the field's efforts to conceptually specify and operationalize the technical strategies and tactics that characterize a particular treatment approach. It must be remembered, however, that the vast majority of treatment manuals has been written by psychotherapy researchers for the purpose of training therapists–subjects to participate in research on treatment, especially outcome studies. We do not know the extent to which treatment manuals are used in formal graduate training programs, nor do we have any data about the impact of manual use in such programs. Therefore, any information we have about the impact of treatment manuals on training comes from the experiences and data of researchers who are only secondarily interested in training.

Post hoc investigations of psychotherapy training, conducted in the context of a manual-based treatment process and/or outcome study, result in several serious methodological problems (Miller & Binder, 2002): (1) format effects, (2) trainer effects, (3) therapist effects, (4) measurement inadequacies, and (5) problematic design features.

Format Effects

Across studies there are no uniform or consistent definitions of manual-based training. Training components and the extent and intensity of training vary enormously across studies.

Trainer Effects

Trainer effects is a seriously neglected issue. There is likely wide variations in teaching skills and effectiveness across trainers, even when the
content is standardized with a manual. In the only two identified studies specifically devoted to studying the outcome of training, trainers
using the same manuals in each study evidenced varying degrees of
effectiveness in conducing technical adherence in their trainees (Hamovitch, 1985; Henry, Strupp, Butler, Schacht, & Binder, 1993).

Therapist Effects

The "Vanderbilt II" study, conducted in the 1980s and led by Hans
Strupp (Strupp, 1993), was designed specifically to examine the impact
of manual-guided training on therapist performance. I was fortunate
to be a part of that research team and collaborate with Strupp in the
development and implementation of the training program. The performance of 16 therapists (licensed clinical psychologists and psychiatrists) was measured prior to, and after, participation in a year-long
training program. We found that variables associated with the therapist-
trainees' prior supervision experiences and with features of their
personalities had an impact on their responses to the training program:
There was an inverse correlation between amount of prior supervision
and adherence to the prescribed techniques of the treatment model being taught; in addition, those therapists who were rated as the most
intensely self-critical tended to evince rigid adherence to prescribed
techniques and more hostile behavior toward their patients (Henry,
Schacht, et al., 1993).

Measurement Inadequacies

The definition of *technical adherence* has always been more precise for
any given treatment model than the definition of *competence*. Still, significant improvement in the uniformity of adherence measures is
needed before extensive cross-study comparisons can be made readily.
Furthermore, our conceptions of *therapeutic competence* need significant
refinement. For example, competence tends to be rated as though it
were a fixed feature of each technical intervention. In fact, therapeutic
competence probably is more validly conceived as a fluid variable that
guides the selection and shaping of interventions in response to immediate contextual exigencies (Binder, 1999).

Problematic Design Features

The designs of most manual-based training programs that are part of treatment outcome studies limit the generalizability of findings to formal graduate training programs and to continuing education formats. The most important limitation of these research designs, however, is the absence of baseline data on therapist performance.

Although there are serious limitations to the validity and generalizability of manual-based training research findings, here are those findings in a nutshell:

1. Manual-based training can produce significant increments in adherence to prescribed therapeutic techniques, but this effect does not produce better treatment outcomes, by itself (Lambert & Okiishi, 1997; Miller & Binder, 2002).

2. The impact of manual-based training on the therapeutic competence of trainees is inconclusive.

3. Technical adherence and therapeutic competence are overlapping but not synonymous phenomena, as inferred from the low correlations between ratings of the two variables. In other words, there is much more to therapeutic competence than using techniques prescribed by a treatment model.

4. There is some evidence that manual-based training within the context of treatment research accelerates the acquisition of prescribed techniques, and perhaps skills, as well as reducing variability in therapist effectiveness (Crits-Christoph & Mintz, 1991; Miller & Binder, 2002). On the other hand, there is also evidence that enormous variability in effectiveness remains across therapists and across patients for a given therapist (again, within the context of manual-based treatment studies; Luborsky et al., 1997). Whether the manual-based treatment is supportive–expressive, or cognitive-behavioral, psychodynamic, or interpersonal, researchers have commented on the noteworthy variability in performance and effectiveness across therapists (Bein et al., 2000; Hollon, 1996; Luborsky et al., 1997; O'Malley et al., 1988).

As far as I know, Vanderbilt II is the only large-scale manual-guided study that has gathered data on therapist performance before as well as after the training. We found that use of a manual-guided didactic seminar, videotaped illustrations of exemplary technique, and several months of small-group supervision of one training case per therapist resulted in significant increments in adherence to techniques prescribed by the model (Henry, Strupp, et al., 1993).

There were, however, untoward training effects. There was a tendency for the therapists' interpersonal performance to deteriorate immediately after training. They tended to take a more adversarial stance toward their posttraining patients. One of the causes of this state of affairs was quite ironic. The treatment model emphasized dealing with the interpersonal management of difficult patients. Consequently, training focused on identification and management of hostile transference and countertransference enactments. I think the training sensitized the therapists to the prospect of hostile attitudes and behavior from their patients but did not, at the same time, give them confidence that they could successfully manage this behavior. As a result, these therapists were warier of their patients after training.

These conjectures were indirectly supported by subsequent analyses and reanalyses of the Vanderbilt II data, which suggested that the therapists did not seem to develop an overall competence in implementing the treatment approach. This finding was reflected in the absence of noticeable enhancement of their therapeutic effectiveness (Bein et al., 2000). In a word, this unique study of the impact of therapy training was far from encouraging. The study was designed to assess the impact of manual-guided training on the performance of experienced therapists. Of course, we do not know if the findings can be generalized to novice clinicians in graduate training programs.

Psychotherapy training needs to be revamped from beginning to end. In the absence of an adequate research-informed pedagogical theory for psychotherapy training, pedagogical concepts and principles that have been formulated through research in the cognitive sciences on the nature and development of skillful performances across various knowledge domains can be adapted to guide the training of psychotherapists (Binder, 1999).

THE PROBLEM OF "INERT" KNOWLEDGE

The novice therapist flounders around for an indefinite period of time. All of that knowledge that has been acquired in course work appears to disappear — or worse, it becomes a distracting jumble of fragmented ideas and rules that disorients rather than guides and that makes it difficult to hear the patient. Cognitive scientists have recognized that novices in all fields go through some period of performance disorientation when learning new techniques and skills (Binder, 1993). The psychotherapy training literature, however, glosses over this phenomenon.

The problem of knowledge transfer begins in the classroom, where psychotherapy principles and procedures, along with their theoretical rationales, are taught. Knowledge acquired through lectures, discussions, and observations of others doing therapy (e.g., via videotaped recordings) is limited to "declarative knowledge" (see Chapter 1).

As discussed in Chapter 1, although declarative knowledge provides an essential foundation for competent practice, it does not provide guidance about when and how to implement concepts, principles, rules, and procedures. Without such guidance, declarative knowledge is not spontaneously accessed when needed in the context of real-world situations, the knowledge remains "inert." Regarding the practice of psychotherapy, a therapist may not be proficient at conducting therapy, no matter how facile his or her discourse about it. In the words of Edgar Levenson (1998), he or she may be a "locker-room expert," who can "talk a good game" but who is an inept player. Declarative knowledge about therapy is insufficient; the therapist must be able to apply this knowledge as a guide for when and how to act. For example, in the Vanderbilt II training study, the therapists could easily discuss the concept of transference and identify evidence of it in the videotaped sessions they observed. While they were actually conducting therapy, however, they were not nearly as proficient at identifying and effectively working with manifestations of transference.

Proficient and expert therapists bring a know-how, an artistry, to their conduct of psychotherapy. They know what to do in actual clinical situations, which indicates their acquisition and refinement of procedural skills (also discussed in Chapter 1). Highly developed procedural skills are associated with the performance of expert practitioners across knowledge domains and are characterized by the following properties:

1. Domain-relevant pattern recognitions, contextual judgments, and relevant actions are carried out spontaneously.
2. These mental processes and actions are carried out without the practitioner necessarily having been aware of learning to do them.
3. The practitioner usually is unable to describe the knowledge

which his or her performance reveals (Sternberg & Horvath, 1999).

An expert's performance is guided by very rich and complex mental working models that allow for planning, execution, appraisal, and modification of their behavior. In addition, experts have a refined sense of which tacit patterns fit best in the current situation, even when the situation is ambiguous (Ericsson, 1996; Sternberg & Horvath, 1999). They also are able to modify their understanding and actions to respond to unique situations effectively. In other words, they can *improvise* (Binder, 1999). In general, experts stand out by excelling in more complex and unusual circumstances (Ericsson, 1996). For example, it is with difficult cases that the more proficient therapists clearly distinguish themselves from their less proficient peers (Lambert & Okiishi, 1997).

Course work leads to the acquisition of declarative knowledge but is insufficient, by itself, to produce procedural knowledge. Procedural knowledge is acquired through *practice* in implementing declarative knowledge in simulated and actual real-world contexts. Practice experiences are the most productive if the declarative knowledge used during practice is optimally organized. In other words, the ease with which declarative knowledge is transformed into useable procedural knowledge is determined, in large measure, by the teaching methods used to convey the declarative knowledge. Unfortunately, there are serious problems in the U.S. educational system. I do not know to what extent these problems exist in the educational systems of other countries. However, in the words of a cognitive scientist who has extensively studied U.S. educational systems: "Schooling in the United States is all too often a mile wide and an inch deep. Fragmentary topics are taught, quickly memorized, tested, and then forgotten. Also, training courses too often consist of so-called theory first and brief practical experiences afterwards" (Lesgold, 2001, p. 965).

I believe that graduate-level training in psychotherapy suffers from this ubiquitous strategy of skimming the surface of knowledge. A major consequence is the problem of inert clinical knowledge, which was recognized but not fully understood by Fenichel, Menninger, and Levenson. Occasionally, there is a call for radical improvements in clinical training. Changes need to be made in the curriculum of clinical training programs that minimize the discontinuities between education and practice. Classroom experiences need to prepare students more effectively for acquiring procedural knowledge, and clinical educators need to become better teachers (Binder, 1993, 1999; Patton, 2000).

IN THE CLASSROOM

Revamping psychotherapy training—overcoming the problem of inert knowledge—should begin in the classroom, where students first learn about treatment models. There is solid empirical evidence that the methods used to convey information about a subject profoundly influence students' degree of understanding as well as accessibility of this knowledge as a practical guide to action (Bransford, Brown, & Cocking, 2000).

Overcoming Preconceptions

The ways in which students understand new information as well as their receptivity to new ideas are deeply influenced by their existing knowledge about the subject and by their preconceptions about the subject. If this existing knowledge is not evaluated, new concepts and information may not be accurately understood and firmly grasped (Bransford et al., 2000). From a study of how children learn in the classroom, there is an amusing anecdote about children who have the preconception that the earth is flat but are taught that it is round. When queried about their new conception of the earth's shape, many of them described it as pie-shaped—demonstrating their creative assimilation of the new information into their old belief. Children are not the only ones who are influenced by their preconceptions about a subject. In courses that I have taught on the topics of psychodynamic theory, therapy, and brief therapy, I have encouraged students to express their views in the first class meeting and thereby unearthed preconceptions that biased them against the course topics. For example, often students enter graduate clinical training with a prior sole exposure to early psychoanalytic theories; consequently, they believe that psychoanalytic theory is too abstract, misunderstands female development, is too preoccupied with sexual issues, and relies solely on interpretation of early childhood experiences as a therapeutic strategy. Similarly, many students enter my brief therapy course convinced that this form of therapy is merely a rationale for insurance companies to deny patients effective therapeutic services that would be costlier. The influence of preconceptions also can be inferred when experienced therapists are exposed to new treatment approaches. As mentioned, in the Vanderbilt II study those therapists who had the most prior therapy supervision were the least receptive to the new learning experiences offered in the study (Henry, Strupp, et al., 1993). It is likely that these therapists had experienced more prior exposure to specific ideas about therapy processes and procedures and therefore had firmer preconceptions about how therapy should be conducted.

The relevant principle is that any course in psychotherapy should begin by addressing the students' preconceptions about the clinical theories and treatment models to be taught. I have no data about how often graduate-level therapy courses begin this way, but I suspect that it is not a widespread pedagogical strategy. If different racial, ethnic, and cultural groups are represented in the student body, these students should be encouraged to verbalize how their backgrounds and heritages influence their views of the topic.

On the other hand, knowledge and skills previously developed can be a bridge to learning new knowledge and skills (Bransford et al., 2000). For example, when students are struggling to understand how to conduct a therapeutic inquiry, I often encourage them to imagine how they would act if they were at dinner with an acquaintance or friend who was sharing a personal problem. The idea is for the student to draw upon interpersonal skills and inquiry techniques developed in personal relationships but not always spontaneously considered relevant to the novel circumstance of a formal therapeutic interaction.

Focusing on "Big Ideas"

In order for declarative knowledge to be an effective foundation for the development of performance skills, it must be organized around basic concepts or "big ideas." The aim is to develop a thorough understanding of the subject matter in a way that transfers across different situations and that guides skillful action (Bransford et al., 2000). Instructors of therapy courses should avoid barraging students with content in the name of comprehensiveness or presenting material according to some superficial organizational principle (e.g., presenting treatment models in chronological order of development). Instead, instructors should consider which information is essential as a foundation for understanding a treatment approach and which basic concepts would be the most effective way of organizing this information. A focus on teaching a smaller selection of essential content and basic concepts along with many concrete illustrative examples, rather than a wider coverage of material, helps students develop a knowledge base that is more likely to translate into an effective procedural guide to action.

Illustrative examples of content and concepts should be organized around sets of circumstances, when they are relevant. This pedagogical strategy facilitates the transformation of declarative into procedural knowledge (Bransford et al., 2000). For example, in a course on psychodynamic approaches to therapy, a wide variety of types of interactions, mental states, and technical interventions can be organized around the interrelated concepts of transference and countertransference. Rather than presenting these concepts in the abstract, they can be presented in the context of understanding what is happening in the videotaped segments of actual therapies. Conceivably, different definitions of transference and countertransference can be used to give alternative meanings to the same videotaped illustrations, thus demonstrating how the concepts guide understanding and action in actual clinical contexts. Such a teaching strategy should help "conditionalize" the concepts of transference and countertransference.

Facilitating the Development of Metacognitive Skills

The development of self-awareness is a high-priority educational objective in most therapy training programs, where it is conceived as the capacity to attune to one's subjective experience, especially affective reactions to patient–therapist interactions. The capacity to track one's own affective reactions and motivations is considered to be a cardinal factor in maintaining a good alliance and in rectifying alliance ruptures as they occur (Safran & Muran, 2000). This particular attribute, however, is one skill (in a broader set of metacognitive skills) that is characteristic of experts in any performance domain. By *metacognitive skills* I mean the ability to monitor one's own performance, including (1) monitoring one's understanding of a problem context and realizing when additional information is required for thorough comprehension; (2) evaluating whether new information is consistent with what is already known; (3) drawing analogies between the new situation and previously encountered situations in order to enhance understanding and guide action; and (4) modifying understanding and action based on error-correcting feedback (Bransford et al., 2000).

The relevant pedagogical principle is that psychotherapy training should reflect a metacognitive approach to instruction, from classroom course work to supervised practice of therapy. A promising strategy for furthering this approach is the use of "formative assessment," in which students are evaluated frequently on their acquisition of circumscribed knowledge and skills, in order to provide frequent feedback about how well they are learning.

WHAT DO WE KNOW ABOUT THE EFFECTIVENESS OF PSYCHOTHERAPY SUPERVISION?

Although classroom course work is essential for acquiring a foundation of factual and theoretical knowledge, supervised conduct of actual therapies is considered to be the most important preparation for independent professional work. The superordinate goals of therapy supervision are to teach students how (1) to conceptualize clinical material, (2) to select and apply therapeutic interventions, (3) to develop professional beliefs and values, and (4) to adhere to ethical standards of conduct (Lambert & Ogles, 1997).

How psychodynamic therapy supervision has been conceived and conducted has changed over the history of psychotherapy, and still there is no consensus about these matters. Once Freud began to develop psychoanalysis, he also began to tackle the issue of how to train people to conduct his therapy. He believed that the most important educational objective was self-awareness, gained through a lengthy personal analysis, in order to remove neurotic blocks to understanding patients' unconscious material. One of the early psychoanalytic training centers, the Budapest Psychoanalytic Institute, formalized Freud's training strategy by combining supervision with trainees' personal analyses. The Berlin Psychoanalytic Institute, on the other hand, separated the two functions of personal analysis and supervision of analytic training cases (Jacobs, David, & Meyer, 1995). The optimal supervisory balance between therapeutic experiences to promote personal growth and didactic experiences to promote technical competence has been a point of controversy ever since those early days.

A crucial problem with psychodynamic supervision, although considered to be a primary activity of therapists and talked about with regularity, is that it has not been examined to an extent commensurate with its importance. For example, in their recent book on psychoanalytic supervision, Frawley-O'Day and Sarnat (2001) point out that there have been only 10 texts, in addition to their book, devoted to the topic. Typically, therapists are not thoroughly trained to conduct supervision. Even if the desire to train is present, no pedagogical theories have been developed to guide such instruction (Binder & Strupp, 1997b; Dewald, 1987; Frawley-O'Day & Sarnat, 2001; Jacobs et al., 1995).

In the absence of a true pedagogy to guide therapy supervision, the vacuum is filled by the clinical concepts, principles, and procedures that are the mental tools with which therapists are familiar and comfortable. The ways in which supervisors conceive of the supervisory process and the roles of trainee and supervisor tend to reflect the models of treatment that they offer. Classical psychoanalytic therapies adhere to a positivist epistemological philosophy, in which the therapist is viewed as an objective scientist who authoritatively deciphers the patient's associations to explain the origins of unconscious conflicts. Accordingly, the supervisor is viewed as an objective scientist and authoritative teacher who helps students understand the true meanings of the clinical material they present and advises them about appropriate interventions. Difficulties in the supervisory relationship are assumed to represent transference patterns carried over by the trainee from his or her therapy to the supervisory relationship. The supervisor is responsible for interpreting this "parallel process" in order to resolve it by fostering trainee self-awareness (Ekstein & Wallerstein, 1972). Supervision conducted in this fashion allows the supervisor to use knowledge and skills with which he or she is quite familiar (Dewald, 1987).

Contemporary forms of psychodynamic treatment increasingly present a postmodern, constructivist epistemology. The therapist is viewed as a co-participant in a collaborative inquiry wherein therapeutic meanings are co-created. Accordingly, the supervisor is viewed as a co-participant who helps trainees create useful meanings for understanding the clinical material and facilitates their development of a personal technical style. Difficulties in the supervisory relationship tend to be viewed as iatrogenic transference–countertransference enactments growing out of the unique dynamics of the supervisory relationship. The supervisor's task is to help the trainee, and him- or herself disentangle these enactments and refine self-awareness skills in the process (Frawley-O'Day & Sarnat, 2001; Safran & Muran, 2000). Here, too, the supervisor is able to rely on his or her clinical skills.

In contemporary discussions of therapy supervision, a premium is placed on fostering self-exploration to develop self-awareness and the specific metacognitive skill of self-monitoring of affective states. Supervisors believe that this learning process requires circumscribed therapeutic interventions to probe trainees' intentions and motives. Because these interventions risk undermining trainees' self-esteem, the establishment and maintenance of a "supervisory alliance" is considered essential. A great deal of attention is devoted to these quasi-therapeutic issues in books on psychodynamic supervision (Frawley-O'Day & Sarnat, 2001; Jacobs et al., 1995). Although the authors of recent books on supervision attempt to address the teaching of technical strategies and tactics, they invariably revert to this familiar territory of encouraging the personal growth of trainees and minimizing their narcissistic injuries.

Indeed, the emphasis on maintaining a good alliance may unwittingly inhibit supervisors from providing error-correcting feedback that is, perhaps, uncomfortable for the trainee to hear but which is essential for the progressive refinement of skills. In a recent study of the supervisory process, the authors observed that an implicit "rule" often is formed: "We have a very nice relationship, and do not want to say or do anything that may make it less pleasant" (Recihelt & Skjerva, 2002, p. 770).

There is an ancient and simple pedagogical theory that has been grafted onto this quasi-therapeutic teaching model of supervision. Therapy supervision has been characterized as a "master–apprentice" relationship, in which the novice therapist learns the trade by spending time with the master. This classic dyad has served as a model for training craftsman for centuries, and it continues to exert some influence in the training of professionals. The apprentice-therapist learns from the master-supervisor through a process of internalizing and identifying with the latter's ways of thinking about clinical material and of conducting therapy. Internalization processes are developmental/clinical concepts with which therapists are familiar and comfortable. The supervisor's role is to provide a model of clinical thinking and action for the trainee to internalize. A crucial activity for psychodynamic supervisors, then, is to verbalize their thought processes about the clinical material presented by trainees and about their reactions to taped recordings of therapy sessions conducted by their students. In a related activity, which is not so readily utilized, supervisors present recordings of therapies that they have conducted and to explicitly recall as much as possible about the thought processes that accompanied their actions.

Unfortunately, relying on the modeling of therapeutic skills and their presumed internalization raises some evident problems and questions. Perhaps the foremost problem is the supervisor's verbalization of his or her therapeutic skills for the trainee. Cognitive science has demonstrated that the knowledge and skills that characterize a competent performer are largely tacit and therefore not readily accessible to conscious reflection and articulation. In other words, the more skillful a therapist is at doing therapy, the less capable he or she may be of verbalizing the mental processes and actions that mediate this skill. Another problem is the chasm that exists between the importance attributed to modeling competently conducted therapy and the readiness of supervisors to actually expose their work to trainees. I suspect that trainees rarely see their supervisors in action. Finally, there is the question of how much time it takes for someone to actually develop skillful complex performances by trying to imitate the thoughts and actions of a teacher.

NOT TRUE

In point of fact, there is minimal data about the processes and outcomes of therapy supervision. Most empirical investigations of supervision involve surveys of the participants' satisfaction with the experience and with each other. Although it is useful to know the reactions of the participants, what *really* matters is whether the experience produces desired changes in the behavior of trainees and patients. Unfortunately, supervisors' abilities to supervise are rarely evaluated objectively (Dewald, 1987; Jacobs et al., 1995), and there is minimal evidence that supervision changes trainees' actions or affects the outcome of therapy during or after supervision (Bein et al., 2000; Beutler, 1997; Lambert & Ogles, 1997). To quote Recihelt and Skjerva (2002) again, "External validation of variables in supervision of significance for therapist development is badly needed, but the scarcity and poor quality of this kind of research is rather disillusioning" (p. 770).

In the Vanderbilt II study, therapists exposed to more structured supervision tended to adhere more closely to technical prescriptions, but their overall competence was not enhanced and their therapies were not significantly more effective after the training (Henry, Schacht, et al., 1993; Bein et al., 2000). In sum, without substantiating evidence, the presumption that supervision produces competent therapists is a myth (Bickman, 1999).

The sparse evidence, direct and indirect, available from psychotherapy research does indicate that more structured teaching, including structured supervision, produces more effective learning than less structured approaches (Bickman, 1999; Binder, 1993; Lambert & Ogles, 1997). For example, in the early 1990s, I put together a set of recommendations for improving therapy training based on input from a number of colleagues involved in manual-guided training and research. There was general consensus that therapy supervision was too unstructured, that course work and practice in conducting therapy should be more systematically integrated, and that tape recordings of therapy sessions—especially videotapes—were the most valid and useful data to use in supervision (Binder et al., 1993). Systematic observations of the two main supervisors in the Vanderbilt II study suggested that a structured approach promoted the acquisition of prescribed techniques more effectively (Henry, Strupp, et al., 1993). The following specific observations were made about structural supervision:

1. Specific learning tasks should be designated during each supervision session (e.g., listening for allusions to transference patterns, identifying and examining inconsistencies in the patient's view of a situation).
2. When watching and/or listening to a tape-recorded segment of a session, the pattern of therapist–patient interactions should be closely examined as a sample of more general interaction patterns in the session and in the therapy as a whole.
3. When watching and/or listening to tape-recorded segments, clinical material should be used to review major concepts and principles. Also, specific questions should be posed for the novice therapist about his or her performance. In addition to the therapist's affective reactions to the patient, the therapist's thought processes—especially his or her immediate understanding of the patient, the therapeutic process, and the rationales for action—should be examined.
4. The trainee should be given precise feedback about his or her actions that acknowledges good performance and constructively critiques problematic or deficient performance.

The provision of precise feedback during training to engage in complex performances is crucial. Cognitive scientists who have studied the development of expertise across various performance domains have discovered that an extended period of "deliberate practice" is essential to the development of expertise, and that world-class expertise takes a minimum of 10 years of such disciplined practice (Ericsson, 1996; Lehman & Ericsson, 1997). "Deliberate practice" has three components: (1) performance of well-defined tasks at an appropriate level of difficulty; (2) informative feedback; and (3) opportunities for repetition and correction of performance errors (Ericsson, 1996; Lehman & Ericsson, 1997). It is interesting that in the professions—such as psychology, medicine, and law — "practice" refers to what the professional person does *after* training; it is the performance for which training is the goal. In other knowledge domains — such as the arts, music, sports, and scientific research, to some extent — practice refers to the structured training activities that *prepare* the novice for professional activities

The typical psychotherapy training program pushes the novice trainee from course work straight into the clinical work of seeing patients. Supervised treatment, however, is an ineffective format for encouraging the structured activities that constitute deliberate practice. First of all, both the novice therapist and the supervisor have a primary responsibility to respond to the therapeutic needs of the patient, so the therapist's activities are determined by exigencies of the moment. This state of affairs means that component therapy skills are engaged in (i.e., practiced) in an unsystematic way. Secondly, in psychodynamic therapy supervision the supervisor does not have an opportunity to provide feedback until some period of time after the trainee's performance with a patient. Consequently, the trainee does not necessarily have an immediate opportunity to modify incorrect actions. When another opportunity arises, the trainee may or may not recognize it. Furthermore, the connections between therapist actions and immediate and ultimate therapeutic outcomes are complex, subtle, and open to alternative understandings — which compounds an already problematic learning environment. It could be argued that with sufficient experience, novice therapists will develop sufficient competence, even if there are serious weaknesses in the typical supervision format. The problem is that the evidence indicates that experience, per se, is only weakly related to level of performance (Beutler, 1997; Ericsson, 1996).

The concert stage is not the best place to first practice basic piano technique; likewise, the therapy session probably is not the best place to first practice basic therapy technique. Supervised treatment is a teaching format best suited for *refining* therapeutic skills and *elaborating* procedural knowledge across more and more clinical situations *after* the initial foundation of declarative knowledge and therapy skill components has been laid. In other words, a teaching format for novice therapists that allows for deliberate practice needs to be developed and incorporated into formal therapy training.

An innovative instructional format that has been used in teaching schoolchildren, called "anchored instruction," could be applied profitably to the design of a practice format for therapists (The Cognition and Technology Group at Vanderbilt, 1997). The defining feature of an anchored instructional setting is that the presentation of knowledge to be taught in a context that is as similar as possible to actual performance conditions, so that students learn to (1) recognize aspects of problems as they appear in reality, (2) practice differentiating relevant from irrelevant information, and (3) practice making intervening and receiving immediate error-correcting feedback that guides subsequent practice interventions. For example, digitized segments of actual therapy sessions (or scripted therapy vignettes portrayed by actors) that illustrate specific types of issues, problems, concepts, and principles could be presented to the trainee. The trainee's reactions to the material as well as his or her hypothetical interventions could be discussed with a practice "coach." In this teaching format, the trainee would have the simultaneous opportunities of acquiring and applying theoretical knowledge, as well as systematically developing and practicing the clinical pattern recognition skills that are fundamental to therapeutic competence. The novice therapist also could begin developing and practicing basic therapeutic strategies and tactics. New computer-generated visual simulation technology offers the potential to develop therapy simulation programs that may afford especially effective practice formats.

So far I have made recommendations for improving psychotherapy training in clinical programs that grant graduate degrees. It is also possible for licensed practitioners to develop practice routines for the purpose of maintaining and/or enhancing their therapeutic skills. World-class performers in sports, music, and the arts return to coaches and teachers throughout their careers to maintain and enhance their skills. Bad habits can creep into the performances of even the elite in any field. Inexplicably, practitioners in the professions are much less likely to engage in this sort of periodic practice. Continuing education courses and workshops have all the major disadvantages of any teaching format that is limited to the acquisition of declarative knowledge.

The established therapist can develop a practice routine by generating videotape recordings or computer digitized recordings of his or her therapy sessions. These clinical materials can be used to practice various therapeutic skills. Probably the best way of engaging in such practice is to obtain the aid of a coach, who can guide the therapist in getting the most out of a practice session. If having a therapy coach is not possible, therapists can arrange to provide peer coaching to each other, in small-group formats. The most important point is that therapists need to find ways to practice their skills, in order to maintain and enhance them over the course of a career.

I would like to end this chapter, and this book, by articulating the most important aim of psychotherapy training. I am referring to the preparation of the novice therapist to use his or her clinical experience to become an *intuitive* therapist. *Webster's* dictionary defines *intuition* as "the immediate knowing or learning of something without the conscious use of reasoning" (*Webster's Twentieth Century Dictionary*, 1979). The British psychoanalyst, Christopher Bollas stated that a therapist needs the intuitive sense of "where to look, what to look at, and how to look at it" (1992, pp. 89–93). I would add that the therapist also needs an intuitive sense of "what to do about it." In the language of the cognitive sciences, I believe Bollas was referring to the acquisition of the ingrained, extensive procedural clinical knowledge that serves as a foundation for the capacity to understand clinical situations deeply and to improvise in a productive way. Donald Winnicott, the eminent Scottish pediatrician and psychoanalyst, reflected upon the development of his intuitive capacities in this way:

> Changes in my work do occur in the course of time and on account of experience. One could compare my position with that of a cellist who first slogs away at *technique* and then actually becomes able to play *music*, taking technique for granted. I am aware of doing this work more easily and with more success than I was able to do it thirty years ago. . . . (1971, p. 6)

Research and observation reveals that Winnicott's assumption that simple time and experience lead to the development of exquisite intuition is not true. I do not know what combination of talent and training contributed to Winnicott's extraordinary therapeutic abilities. But the challenge for psychotherapy trainers and researchers is to develop training methods that prepare novice therapists more effectively to *play beautiful therapeutic music*.

Epilogue

Over the past three decades, I have had the opportunity to become familiar with the work of many proficient and expert therapists. I have observed several similarities in the way they work or talk about their work. First, these wise therapists tend to focus on the current, major psychological and interpersonal issues that are affecting their patients' everyday lives. Second, they tend to engage their patients in more reciprocal discussions than their less experienced and proficient colleagues, who tend to take a more standard, passive approach. Third, these discussions are characterized by more questions and suggestions than their less experienced and proficient colleagues, who tend to take a more standard interpretive stance. Fourth, more experienced and proficient therapists use more self-disclosure that is in their patients' best interests. Such self-disclosure includes not only the more commonly accepted metacommunications about affective reactions to immediate patient–therapist interactions, but also anecdotes from their personal and professional experiences. Such anecdotes are used to make a point, to educate patients about some aspect of the way they are conducting their lives. Finally, these therapists use these methods of interacting with their patients to improvise approaches that they believe will be the most effective, given the specific circumstances characterizing this particular therapeutic dyad.

The therapeutic methods I have enumerated here reflect the gradual evolution of exceptionally good therapists from technicians, which is what they are taught to be in clinical training programs, to mentors.

Exceptionally good, experienced therapists share their wisdom about life; they mentor and coach their patients as well as interpreting the hidden or obscure meanings of patient actions. This mentoring facet of a therapist's role grows larger as the therapist ages and accumulates increasingly more personal and professional experiences. The highly experienced therapists are able to find parallels between their experiences and an increasingly wide variety of current situations encountered by their patients. I believe this evolution into the role of a mentor explains another observation made about experienced and expert therapists: Across different therapy approaches, the best therapists from all of these approaches conduct therapy in ways more similar to each other than to the less proficient representatives of their own approaches. There is an important implication to be drawn from this observation: One important requisite for improving the training of psychotherapists is to devote at least as much time to identifying and studying the unique features of experienced, expert therapists as is currently spent comparing the effects of different treatment protocols.

In this book I have attempted to encourage just such a point of view: one that puts the mental processes and actions that characterize a proficient therapist in the foreground, and puts the theory-bound technical strategies and tactics in the background. This approach reflects not only my view of good therapy but also the view and life's work of my colleague, mentor, and friend, Hans H. Strupp. The book on time-limited dynamic psychotherapy that we published in 1984 reflected our cumulative experiences conducting and studying psychotherapy up to that time. We knew that it represented a snapshot of knowledge that was always moving—that is, evolving and expanding. What I have presented here represents another snapshot, capturing my view—at this moment in time—of the continuing evolution of our knowledge about psychotherapy.

References

Abend, S. (1995). Discussion of Jay Greenberg's paper on self-disclosure. *Contemporary Psychoanalysis, 31*, 207–211.

Addis, M. E. (1997). Evaluating the treatment manual as a means of disseminating empirically validated psychotherapies. *Clinical Psychology: Science and Practice, 4*, 1–11.

Alexander, F., & French, T. (1946). *Psychoanalytic Therapy: Principles and Applications*. New York: Basic Books.

American Psychiatric Association. (1994). *Diagnostic and Statistical Manual of Mental Disorders* (4th ed.). Washington, DC: Author.

American Psychiatric Association. (2000). *Diagnostic and Statistical Manual of Mental Disorders* (4th ed., text rev.). Washington, DC: Author.

Applebaum, S. A. (1975). Parkinson's Law in psychotherapy. *International Journal of Psychoanalytic Psychotherapy, 4*, 426–436.

Armstrong, S. (1980). Dual focus in brief psychodynamic psychotherapy. *Psychotherapy and Psychosomatics, 33*, 147–154.

Balint, M., Ornstein, P. H., & Balint, E. (1972). *Focal Psychotherapy: An Example of Applied Psychoanalysis*. Philadelphia: Lippincott.

Barber, J. P., Crits-Christoph, P., & Luborsky, L. (1996). Effects of therapist adherence and competence on patient outcome in brief dynamic psychotherapy. *Journal of Consulting and Clinical Psychology, 64*, 619–622.

Barber, J. P., Foltz, C., De Rubeis, R. J., & Landis, J. R. (2002). Consistency of interpersonal themes in narratives about relationships. *Psychotherapy Research, 12*, 139–158.

Barkham, M., Rees, A., Stiles, W. B., Shapiro, D. A., Hardy, G. E., & Reynold, S. (1996). Dose–effect relations in time-limited psychotherapy for depression. *Journal of Consulting and Clinical Psychology, 64*, 927–935.

Barlow, D. H., & Cerny, J. A. (1988). *Psychological Treatment of Panic.* New York: Guilford Press.

Beck, A. T., & Emery, G. (1985). *Anxiety Disorders and Phobias: A Cognitive Perspective.* New York: Basic Books.

Beck, A. T., Rush, J. A., Shaw, B. F., & Emery, G. (1979). *Cognitive Therapy of Depression.* New York: Guilford Press.

Beebe, B., Lachmann, F., & Jaffe, J. (1997). Mother–infant interaction structures and presymbolic self- and object-representations. *Psychoanalytic Dialogues, 7,* 133–187.

Bein, E., Anderson, T., Strupp, H. H., Henry, W. P., Schacht, T. E., Binder, J. L., & Butler, S. F. (2000). The effects of training in time-limited dynamic psychotherapy: Changes in therapeutic outcome. *Psychotherapy Research, 10,* 119–132.

Benjamin, L. S. (1993). *Interpersonal Diagnosis and Treatment of Personality Disorders.* New York: Guilford Press.

Bergin, A. E., & Garfield, L. S. (Eds.). (1994). *Handbook of Psychotherapy and Behavior Change* (4th ed.). New York: Wiley.

Beutler, L. E. (1997). The psychotherapist as a neglected variable in psychotherapy: An illustration by reference to the role of therapist experience and training. *Clinical Psychology: Science and Practice, 4,* 44–52.

Beutler, L. E., & Harwood, T. M. (2000). *Prescriptive Psychotherapy: A Practical Guide to Systematic Treatment Selection.* Oxford, UK: Oxford University Press.

Beutler, L. E., Machado, P. P., & Neufeldt, S. A. (1994). Therapist variables. In A. E. Bergin & S. L. Garfield (Eds.), *Handbook of Psychotherapy and Behavior Change* (4th ed., pp. 229–269). New York: Wiley.

Bickman, L. (1999). Practice makes perfect and other myths about mental health services. *American Psychologist, 54,* 965–978.

Binder, J. L. (1993). Is it time to improve psychotherapy training? *Clinical Psychology Review, 13,* 301–318.

Binder, J. L. (1999). Issues in teaching and learning time-limited dynamic psychotherapy. *Clinical Psychology Review, 19,* 705–719.

Binder, J. L., Henry, W. P., & Strupp, H. H. (1987). An appraisal of selection criteria for dynamic psychotherapies and implications for setting time limits. *Psychiatry: Journal for the Study of Interpersonal Processes, 50,* 154–166.

Binder, J. L., & Strupp, H. H. (1991). The Vanderbilt approach to time-limited dynamic psychotherapy. In P. Crits-Christoph & J. Barber (Eds.), *Handbook of Short-Term Dynamic Therapy* (pp. 137–165). New York: Basic Books.

Binder, J. L., & Strupp, H. H. (1997a). "Negative process": A recurrently discovered and underestimated facet of therapeutic process and outcome in the individual psychotherapy of adults. *Clinical Psychology: Science and Practice, 4,* 121–139.

Binder, J. L., & Strupp, H. H. (1997b). Supervision in psychodynamic psychotherapies. In C. E. Watkins, Jr. (Ed.), *Handbook of Psychotherapy Supervision* (pp. 44–62). New York: Wiley.

Binder, J. L., Strupp, H. H., Bongar, B., Lee, S. L., Messer, S., & Peakes, T. H. (1993). Recommendations for improving psychotherapy training based on experiences with manual-guided training and research: Epilogue. *Psychotherapy, 30,* 599–600.

Blatt, S. J., Sanislow, C. A, Zuroff, D. C., & Pilkonis, P. A. (1996). Characteristics of effective therapists: Further analysis of data from the National Institute of Mental Health treatment of depression collaborative research program. *Journal of Consulting and Clinical Psychology, 64,* 1276–1284.

Bohart, A. C., O'Hara, M., & Leitner, L. M. (1988). Empirically violated treatments: Disenfranchisement of humanistic and other psychotherapies. *Psychotherapy Research, 8,* 141–157.

Bollas, C. (1992). *Being and Character: Psychoanalysis and Self Experience.* New York: Hill & Wang.

Book, H. E. (1998). *How to Practice Brief Psychodynamic Psychotherapy: The Core Conflict Relationship Theme Method.* Washington, DC: American Psychological Association.

Bowlby, J. (1969). *Attachment and Loss: Vol. I. Attachment.* New York: Basic Books.

Bowlby, J. (1988). *A Secure Base: Parent–Child Attachment and Human Development.* New York: Basic Books.

Bransford, J. D., Brown, A. L., & Cocking, R. R. (2000). *How People Learn: Brain, Mind, Experience, and School.* Washington, DC: National Academy Press.

Bransford, J. D., Franks, J. J., Vye, N. J., & Sherwood, R. D. (1989). New approaches to instruction: Because wisdom can't be told. In S. Vosniadou & A. Ortony (Eds.), *Similarity and Analogical Reasoning* (pp. 470–497). New York: Cambridge University Press.

Budman, S. H., & Gurman, A. S. (1988). *Theory and Practice of Brief Therapy.* New York: Guilford Press.

Chambless, D. L., & Hollon, S. D. (1998). Defining empirically supported therapies. *Journal of Clinical and Consulting Psychology, 66,* 7–18.

Chambless, D. L., & Ollendick, T. H. (2001). Empirically supported psychological interventions: Controversies and evidence. *Annual Review of Psychology, 52,* 685–716.

Chi, M. T., Glaser, R., & Farr, M. J. (Eds.). (1988). *The Nature of Expertise.* Hillsdale, NJ: Erlbaum.

Christensen, A., & Jacobson, N. S. (1994). Who (or what) can do psychotherapy?: The status and challenge of nonprofessional therapies. *Psychological Science, 5,* 8–14.

Cognition and Technology Group at Vanderbilt, The. (1997). *The Jasper Project: Lessons in Curriculum, Instruction, Assessment, and Professional Development.* Mahwah, NJ: Erlbaum.

Cohen, M. S., Freeman, J. T., & Wolf, S. (1996). Metarecognition in time-stressed decision making: Recognizing, critiquing, and correcting. *Human Factors, 38,* 206–219.

Connolly, M. B., Crits-Christoph, P., Barber, J. P., & Luborsky, L. (2000). Transference patterns in the therapeutic relationship in supportive–expressive psychotherapy for depression. *Psychotherapy Research, 10,* 356–372.

Connolly, M. B., Crits-Christoph, P., Demorest, A., Azarian, K., Muenz, L., & Chittams, J. (1996). Varieties of transference patterns in psychotherapy. *Journal of Consulting and Clinical Psychology, 64,* 1213–1221.

Connolly, M. B., Crits-Christoph, P., Shappell, S., Barber, J. P., & Luborsky, L. (1998). Therapist interventions in early sessions of brief supportive–expressive psychotherapy for depression. *Journal of Psychotherapy Practice and Research, 7*, 290–300.

Connolly, M. B., Crits-Christoph, P., Shappell, S., Barber, J. P., Luborsky, L., & Shaffer, C. (1999). Relation of transference interpretations to outcome in the early sessions of brief supportive–expressive psychotherapy. *Psychotherapy Research, 9*, 485–495.

Connolly-Gibbons, M. B., Crits-Christoph, P., de la Cruz, C., Barber, J. P., Siqueland, L., & Gladis, M. (2003). Pretreatment expectations, interpersonal functioning, and symptoms in the prediction of the therapeutic alliance across supportive–expressive psychotherapy and cognitive therapy. *Psychotherapy Research, 13*, 59–76.

Crits-Christoph, P. (1998). The interpersonal interior of psychotherapy. *Psychotherapy Research, 8*, 1–16.

Crits-Christoph, P., Barber, J. P., & Kurcias, J. C. (1993). The accuracy of therapists' interpretations and the development of the therapeutic alliance. *Psychotherapy Research, 3*, 25–35.

Crits-Christoph, P., Connolly, M. B., Shappell, S., Elkin, I., Krupnick, J., & Sotsky, S. (1999). Interpersonal narratives in cognitive and interpersonal psychotherapies. *Psychotherapy Research, 9*, 22–35.

Crits-Christoph, P., & Connolly-Gibbons, M. B. (2001). Relational interpretations. *Psychotherapy: Theory, Research, Practice, Training, 38*, 423–428.

Crits-Christoph, P., Cooper, A., & Luborsky, L. (1988). The accuracy of therapists' interpretations and the outcome of dynamic psychotherapy. *Journal of Consulting and Clinical Psychology, 56*, 490–495.

Crits-Christoph, P., Demorest, A., Muenz, R. R., & Baranackie, K. (1994). Consistency of interpersonal themes for patients in psychotherapy. *Journal of Personality, 62*, 499–526.

Crits-Christoph, P., & Mintz, J. (1991). Implications of therapist effects for the design and analysis of comparative studies of psychotherapies. *Journal of Consulting and Clinical Psychology, 59*, 20–26.

Cummings, N., & Sayama, M. (1995). *Focused Psychotherapy: A Casebook of Brief, Intermittent Psychotherapy Throughout the Life Cycle*. New York: Brunner/Mazel.

Davanloo, H. B. (1980). *Short-Term Dynamic Psychotherapy*. New York: Aronson.

Della Selva, P. C. (1996). *Intensive Short-Term Dynamic Psychotherapy: Theory and Technique*. New York: Wiley.

Detrie, T., & McDonald, M. C. (1997). Managed care and the future of psychiatry. *Archives of General Psychiatry, 54*, 201–204.

Dewald, P. (1987). *Learning Processes in Psychoanalytic Supervision: Complexities and Challenges*. Madison, CT: International Universities Press.

Dreyfus, H. L., & Dreyfus, S. E. (1988). *Mind over Machine: The Power of Human Intuition and Expertise in the Era of the Computer*. New York: Free Press.

Eagle, M. N., & Wolitzky, D. L. (1992). Psychoanalytic theories of psychotherapy. In D. K. Freedheim (Eds.), *History of Psychotherapy: A Century of Change* (pp. 109–158). Washington, DC: American Psychological Association.

Eells, T. D. (Ed.). (1997). *Handbook of Psychotherapy Case Formulation*. New York: Guilford Press.

Ekstein, R., & Wallerstein, R. S. (1972). *The Teaching and Learning of Psychotherapy* (rev. ed.). Oxford, UK: International Universities Press.

Elstein, A. S. (1997, June–July). *Training of clinical reasoning processes in medicine*. Paper presented at the conference on The Training of Psychotherapist's Information Processing in the Future, Grindelwald, Switzerland.

Epstein, L. (1995). Self-disclosure and analytic space. *Contemporary Psychoanalysis, 31*, 229–236.

Ericsson, K. A. (Ed.). (1996). *The Road to Excellence: The Acquisition of Expert Performance in the Arts and Sciences, Sports and Games*. Mahwah, NJ: Erlbaum.

Ericsson, K. A., & Charness, N. (1999). Expert performance: Its structure and acquisition. In S. J. Ceci & W. M. Williams (Eds.), *The Nature–Nurture Debate: The Essential Readings* (pp. 199–255). Malden, MA: Blackwell.

Fairbairn, W. R. D. (1952). *An Object Relations Theory of Personality*. New York: Basic Books.

Feltovich, P. J., Ford, K. M., & Hoffman, R. R. (Eds.). (1997). *Expertise in Context: Human and Machine*. Cambridge, MA: MIT Press.

Fenichel, O. (1941). *Problems of Psychoanalytic Technique*. Albany, NY: Psychoanalytic Quarterly.

Ferenczi, S., & Rank, O. (1925). *The Development of Psychoanalysis*. New York: Nervous and Mental Disease Publishing.

Firestein, S. K. (2001). *Termination in Psychoanalysis and Psychotherapy* (rev. ed.). Madison, WI: International Universities Press.

Fonagy, P., Steele, M., & Steele, H. (1995). Attachment, the reflective self, and borderline states: The predictive specificity of the Adult Attachment Interview and pathological emotional development. In S. Goldberg & R. Muir (Eds.), *Attachment Theory: Social, Developmental, and Clinical Perspectives* (pp. 233–278). Hillsdale, NJ: Analytic Press.

Foreman, S., & Marmar, C. R. (1995). Therapist actions that address initially poor alliances in psychotherapy. *American Journal of Psychiatry, 142*, 922–926.

Frank, K. A. (1999). *Psychoanalytic Participation*. Hillsdale, NJ: Analytic Press.

Frawley-O'Day, M. G., & Sarnat, J. E. (2001). *The Supervisory Relationship: A Contemporary Psychodynamic Approach*. New York: Guilford Press.

Freud, S. (1955). The psychotherapy of hysteria. In *Standard Edition* (Vol. 2, pp. 255–303). London: Hogarth Press. (Original work published 1893–1895)

Freud, S. (1955). The dynamics of transference. In *Standard Edition* (Vol. 12, pp. 99–108). London: Hogarth Press. (Original work published 1912)

Fridrum, W., Coyle, A., & Lyons, E. (1999). How counseling psychologists view their personal therapy. *British Journal of Medical Psychology, 72*, 545–555.

Gabbard, G. O., Horwitz, L., Allen, J. G., Frieswyk, S., Newsom, G., Colson, D. B., & Coyne, L. (1994). Transference interpretations in the psychotherapy of borderline patients: A high-risk, high-gain phenomenon. *Harvard Review of Psychiatry, 2*, 59–69.

Garfield, S. L. (1990). Issues and methods in psychotherapy research. *Journal of Consulting and Clinical Psychology, 58*, 273–280.

Garfield, S. L. (1994). Research on client variables in psychotherapy. In A. E.

Bergin & S. L. Garfield (Eds.). *Handbook of Psychotherapy and Behavior Change* (4th ed., pp. 190–228). New York: Wiley.

Garfield, S. L. (1997). The therapist as a neglected variable in psychotherapy research. *Clinical Psychology: Science and Practice, 4,* 40–43.

Garfield, S. L. (1998). *The Practice of Brief Psychotherapy.* New York: Wiley.

Glaser, R. (1989). Expertise and learning: How do we think about instructional processes now that we have discovered knowledge structures. In D. Klahr & K. Kotovsky (Eds.), *Complex Information Processing: The Impact of Herbert A. Simon* (pp. 269–282). Hillsdale, NJ: Erlbaum.

Glaser, R., & Chi, M. T. (1988). Overview. In M. T. Chi, R. Glaser, & M. J. Farr (Eds.), *The Nature of Expertise* (pp. xv–xxviii). Hillsdale, NJ: Erlbaum.

Gill, M. M. (1982). *Analysis of Transference: Vol. I. Theory and Technique.* New York: International Universities Press.

Goldberg, C. (1992). *The Seasoned Psychotherapist: Triumph over Adversity.* New York: Norton.

Goldfried, M. R., Raue, P. J., & Castonguay, L. G. (1998). The therapeutic focus in significant sessions of master therapists: A comparison of cognitive–behavioral and psychodynamic-interpersonal interventions. *Journal of Consulting and Clinical Psychology, 66,* 803–810.

Greenberg, J. (1995). Self-disclosure: Is it psychoanalysis? *Contemporary Psychoanalysis, 31,* 193–205.

Greenberg, J. R., & Mitchell, S. A. (1983). *Object Relations in Psychoanalytic Theory.* Cambridge, MA: Harvard University Press.

Greenson, R. (1967). *The Technique and Practice of Psychoanalysis* (Vol. 1). Madison, WI: International Universities Press.

Greenson, R. R., & Wexler, M. (1969). The nontransference relationship in the psychoanalytic situation. *International Journal of Psychoanalysis, 50,* 27–39.

Groopman, J. (2000). *Second Opinions.* New York: Viking.

Gustafson, J. P. (1995). *Brief versus Long Psychotherapy.* Northvale, NJ: Aronson.

Hamilton, N. G. (1988). *Self and Others. Object Relations Theory in Practice.* Northvale, NJ: Aronson.

Hamovitch, G. (1985). An evaluation of competency-based training in short-term dynamic psychotherapy. *Dissertation Abstracts International, 45,* 3071.

Hardy, G. E., Aldridge, J. Davidson, C., Rowe, C., Reilly, S., & Shapiro, D. A. (1999). Therapist responsiveness to client attachment styles and issues observed in client-identified significant events in psychodynamic–interpersonal psychotherapy. *Psychotherapy Research, 9,* 36–53.

Hatcher, S. L., Huebner, D. A., & Zakin, D. F. (1986). Following the trail of the focus in time-limited psychotherapy. *Psychotherapy, 23,* 513–520.

Henry, W. P., Schacht, T. E., & Strupp, H. H. (1986). Structural analysis of social behavior: Application to a study of interpersonal process in differential psychotherapeutic outcome. *Journal of Consulting and Clinical Psychology, 54,* 27–31.

Henry, W. P., Schacht, T. E., Strupp, H. H., Butler, S. F., & Binder, J. L. (1993). Effects of training in time-limited dynamic psychotherapy: Changes in therapist behavior. *Journal of Consulting and Clinical Psychology, 61,* 434–440.

Henry, W. P., & Strupp, H. H. (1994). The therapeutic alliance as interpersonal process. In A. O. Horvath & L. S. Greenberg (Eds.), *The Working Alliance: Theory, Research and Practice* (pp. 51–84). New York: Wiley.

Henry, W. P., Strupp, H. H., Butler, S. F., Schacht, T. E., & Binder, J. L. (1993). Effects of training in time-limited dynamic psychotherapy: Mediators of therapists' responses to training. *Journal of Consulting and Clinical Psychology, 61,* 441–447.

Henry, W. P., Strupp, H. H., Schacht, T. E., & Gaston, L. (1994). Psychodynamic approaches. In A. E. Bergin & S. L. Garfield (Eds.), *Handbook of Psychotherapy and Behavior Change* (4th ed., pp. 143–189). New York: Wiley.

Hill, C. E., & Knox, S. (2001). Self-disclosure. *Psychotherapy, 38,* 413–417.

Hoffman, I. Z. (1983). The patient as interpreter of the analyst's experience. *Contemporary Psychoanalysis, 19,* 389–422.

Hoglend, P. (1996). Analysis of transference in patients with personality disorders. *Journal of Personality Disorders, 10,* 122–131.

Hoglend, P. (2003). Long-term effects of brief dynamic psychotherapy. *Psychotherapy Research, 13,* 271–292.

Hoglend, P., & Piper, W. E. (1995). Focal adherence in brief dynamic psychotherapy: A comparison of findings from two independent studies. *Psychotherapy, 32,* 618–628.

Hoglend, P., Sorlie, T., Heyerdahl, O., Sorbye, O., & Amlo, S. (1993). Brief dynamic psychotherapy: Patient suitability, treatment length, and outcome. *The Journal of Psychotherapy Practice and Research, 2,* 230–241.

Hollon, S. D. (1996). The efficacy and effectiveness of psychotherapy relative to medications. *American Psychologist, 51,* 1025–1030.

Hollon, S. D., & Beck, A. T. (2004). Cognitive and Cognitive Behavioral Therapies. In M. J. Lambert (Ed.), *Bergin and Garfield's Handbook of Psychotherapy and Behavior Change* (5th ed., pp. 447–492). New York: Wiley.

Holyoak, K. J. (1991). Symbolic connectionism: Toward third-generation theories of expertise. In K. A. Ericsson & J. Smith (Eds.), *Toward a General Theory of Expertise* (pp. 301–335). New York: Cambridge University Press.

Horowitz, M. J. (1998). *Cognitive Psychodynamics: From Conflict to Character.* New York: Wiley.

Horvath, A. O. (2001). The alliance. *Psychotherapy: Theory, Research, Practice, Training, 38,* 365–372.

Horvath, A. O., & Greenberg, L. S. (1994). *The Working Alliance: Theory, Research, and Practice.* New York: Wiley.

Howard, K. I., Kopta, S. M., Krause, M. S., & Orlinsky, D. E. (1986). The dose–effect relationship in psychotherapy. *American Psychologist, 41,* 159–164.

Hoyt, M. F. (1979). Aspects of termination in time-limited brief psychotherapy. *Psychiatry, 42,* 208–219.

Ivey, A. E. (1971). *Microcounseling: Innovations in interviewing training.* Oxford, UK: Charles C. Thomas.

Jacobs, D., David, P., & Meyer, D. (1995). *The Supervisory Encounter.* Oxford, UK: Charles C. Thomas.

Johnson, M. E., Papp, C., Schacht, T. E., Mellon, J., & Strupp, H. H. (1989). Converging evidence for identification of recurrent relationship themes: Comparison of two methods. *Psychiatry, 52,* 275–288.

Kavanagh, G. (1995). Process of therapeutic action and change. In M. Lionells, J. Fiscalini, C. H. Mann, & D. B. Stern (Eds.), *Handbook of Interpersonal Psychoanalysis* (pp. 569–602). Hillsdale, NJ: Analytic Press.

Kazdin, A. E. (2000). Evaluating the impact of clinical psychology training programs: Process and outcome issues. *Clinical Psychology: Science and Practice, 7,* 357–360.

Kernberg, O. (1984). *Severe Personality Disorders: Psychotherapeutic Strategies.* New Haven, CT: Yale University Press.

Kiesler, D. J. (1966). Some myths of psychotherapy research and the search for a paradigm. *Psychological Bulletin, 65,* 110–136.

Kiesler, D. J. (1996). *Contemporary Interpersonal Theory and Research: Personality, Psychopathology, and Psychotherapy.* New York: Wiley.

Kihlstrom, J. F. (1987). The cognitive unconscious. *Science, 237,* 1445–1452.

Klerman, G. L., Weissman, M. M., Rounsaville, B. J., & Chevron, E. S. (1984). *Interpersonal Psychotherapy of Depression.* New York: Basic Books.

Kopta, S. M., Howard, K. I., Lowry, J. L., & Beutler, L. E. (1994). Patterns of symptomatic recovery in psychotherapy. *Journal of Consulting and Clinical Psychology, 62,* 1009–1016.

Koss, M. P., & Shiang, J. (1994). Research on brief psychotherapy. In A. E. Bergin & S. L. Garfield (Eds.), *Handbook of Psychotherapy and Behavior Change* (4th ed., pp. 664–700). New York: Wiley.

Lambert, M. J. (2003). *Bergin and Garfield's Handbook of Psychotherapy and Behavior Change* (5th ed.). New York: Wiley.

Lambert, M. J., & Bergin, A E. (1994). The effectiveness of psychotherapy. In A E. Bergin & S. L. Garfield (Eds.), *Handbook of Psychotherapy and Behavior Change* (4th ed., pp. 143–189). New York: Wiley.

Lambert, M. J., Hansen, N. B., & Finch, A. E. (2001). Patient-focused research: Using patient outcome data to enhance treatment effects. *Journal of Consulting and Clinical Psychology, 69,* 159–172.

Lambert, M. J., & Ogles, B. M. (1997). The effectiveness of psychotherapy supervision. In C. E. Watkins, Jr. (Ed.), *Handbook of Psychotherapy Supervision* (pp. 421–446). New York: Wiley.

Lambert, M. J., & Ogles, B. M. (2004). The efficacy and effectiveness of psychotherapy. In M. J. Lambert (Ed.), *Bergin and Garfield's Handbook of Psychotherapy and Behavior Change* (5th ed., pp. 139–193). New York: Wiley.

Lambert, M. J., & Okiishi, J. C. (1997). The effects of the individual psychotherapist and implications for future research. *Clinical Psychology: Science and Practice, 4,* 66–75.

Lambert, M. J., Whipple, J. L., Smart, D. W., Vermeersch, D. A., Nielsen, S. L., & Hawkings, E. J. (2001). The effects of providing therapists with feedback on patient progress during psychotherapy: Are outcomes enhanced? *Psychotherapy Research, 11,* 49–68.

Lambert, M. J., Whipple, J. L., Vermeersch, D. A., Smart, D. W., Hawkins, E. J., Nielsen, S. L., & Goates, M. (2002). Enhancing psychotherapy outcomes via providing feedback on client progress: A replication. *Clinical Psychology and Psychotherapy, 9,* 91–103.

Lansford, E. (1986). Weakenings and repairs of the working alliance in short-term psychotherapy. *Professional Psychology: Research and Practice, 17,* 364–366.

Lazarus, A. A., & Messer, S. B. (1991). Does chaos prevail? An exchange on technical eclecticism and assimilative integration. *Journal of Psychotherapy Integration, 1,* 143–158.

Lehman, A. C., & Ericsson, K. (1997). Research on expert performance and deliberate practice: Implication for the education of amateur musicians and music students. *Psychomusicology, 16,* 40–58.

Lesgold, A. M. (2001). The nature and methods of learning by doing. *American Psychologist, 56,* 964–973.

Levenson, E. A. (1972). *The Fallacy of Understanding: An Inquiry into the Changing Structure of Psychoanalysis.* New York: Basic Books.

Levenson, E. A. (1985). The interpersonal (Sullivanian) model. In A. Rothstein (Ed.), *Models of the Mind* (pp. 49–67). New York: International Universities Press.

Levenson, E. A. (1988). The pursuit of the particular: On the psychoanalytic inquiry. *Contemporary Psychoanalysis, 24,* 1–16.

Levenson, E. A. (1998). Awareness, insight, and learning. *Contemporary Psychoanalysis, 34,* 239–249.

Levenson, H. (1995). *Time-Limited Dynamic Psychotherapy: A Guide to Clinical Practice.* New York: Basic Books.

Levenson, H., Butler, S. F., & Beitman, B. D. (1997). *Concise Guide to Brief Dynamic Psychotherapy.* Washington, DC: American Psychiatric Press.

Levenson, H., & Strupp, H. H. (1997). Cyclical maladaptive patterns: Case formulation in time-limited dynamic psychotherapy. In T. D. Eells (Ed.), *Handbook of Psychotherapy Case Formulation* (pp. 84–115). New York: Guilford Press.

Luborsky, L. (1984). *Principles of Psychoanalytic Psychotherapy: A Manual for Supportive–Expressive Treatment.* New York: Basic Books.

Luborsky, L. (1997a). The core conflict relationship theme: A basic case formulation method. In T. D. Eells (Ed.), *Handbook of Psychotherapy Case Formulation* (pp. 58–83). New York: Guilford Press.

Luborsky, L. (1997b). The convergence of Freud's observations about transference and the CCRT evidence. In L. Luborsky & P. Crits-Christoph, *Understanding Transference: The Core Conflict Relationship Theme Method* (2nd ed., pp. 307–325). Washington, DC: American Psychological Association.

Luborsky, L., & Crits-Christoph, P. (1997). *Understanding Transference: The Core Conflict Relationship Theme Method* (2nd ed.). Washington, DC: American Psychological Association.

Luborsky, L., & De Rubeis, R. J. (1984). The use of psychotherapy manuals: A small revolution in psychotherapy research style. *Clinical Psychology Review, 4,* 5–14.

Luborsky, L., McClellan, A. T., Diguer, L., Woody, G., & Seligman, D. A. (1997). The psychotherapist matters: Comparison of outcomes across twenty-two therapists and seven patient samples. *Clinical Psychology: Science and Practice, 4,* 53–65.

Lyddon, W. J. (1995). Forms and facets of constructivist psychology. In R. A.

Neimeyer & M. J. Mahoney (Eds.), *Constructivism in Psychotherapy* (pp. 69–92). Washington, DC: American Psychological Association.

Macran, S., & Shapiro, D. A. (1998). The role of personal therapy for therapists: A review. *British Journal of Medical Psychology, 7,* 13–25.

Madill, A., & Barkham, M. (1997). Discourse analysis of a theme in one successful case of brief psychodynamic–interpersonal psychotherapy. *Journal of Counseling Psychology, 44,* 232–244.

Magnavita, J. J. (1997). *Restructuring Personality Disorders: A Short-Term Dynamic Approach.* New York: Guilford Press.

Mahler, M. S., Pine, F., & Bergman, A. (1970). The mother's reaction to her toddler's drive for individuation. In E. J. Anthony & T. Benedek (Eds.), *Parenthood: Its Psychology and Psychopathology* (pp. 257–274). Boston: Little, Brown.

Malan, D. H. (1976a). *The Frontier of Brief Psychotherapy.* New York: Plenum Press.

Malan, D. H. (1976b). *Toward the Validation of Dynamic Psychotherapy: A Replication.* New York: Plenum Press.

Malan, D. H. (1979). *Individual Psychotherapy and the Science of Psychodynamics.* London: Butterworths.

Mann, J. (1973). *Time-Limited Psychotherapy.* Cambridge, MA: Harvard University Press.

Mann, J., & Goldman, R. (1982). *A Casebook in Time-Limited Psychotherapy.* New York: McGraw-Hill.

Martin, D. J., Garske, J. P., & Davis, M. K. (2000). Relation of the therapeutic alliance with outcome and other variables: A meta-analytic review. *Journal of Consulting and Clinical Psychology, 68,* 438–450.

Marx, J. A., & Gelso, C. J. (1987). Termination in individual counseling in a university counseling center. *Journal of Counseling Psychology, 34,* 3–9.

Marziali, E. A. (1984). Prediction of outcome of brief psychotherapy from therapist interpretive interventions. *Archives of General Psychiatry, 41,* 301–304.

Menninger, K. (1958). *Theory of Psychoanalytic Technique.* Oxford, England: Basic Books.

Menninger, K., & Holzman, P. S. (1973). *Theory of Psychoanalytic Technique.* New York: Basic Books.

Messer, S. B. (1992). A critical examination of belief structures in integrative and eclectic psychotherapy. In J. C. Norcross & M. R. Goldfried (Eds.), *Handbook of Psychotherapy Integration* (pp. 130–165). New York: Basic Books.

Messer, S. B., Tishby, O., & Spillman, A. (1992). Taking context seriously in psychotherapy research: Relating therapist interventions to patient progress in brief psychoanalytic therapy. *Journal of Consulting and Clinical Psychology, 60,* 678–688.

Messer, S. B., & Warren, C. S. (1995). *Models of Brief Psychodynamic Therapy: A Comparative Approach.* New York: Guilford Press.

Messer, S. B., & Wolitzky, D. L. (1997). The traditional psychoanalytic approach to case formulation. In E. D. Eells (Ed.), *Handbook of Psychotherapy Case Formulation* (pp. 26–57). New York: Guilford Press.

McCullough, L., & Andrews, S. (2001). Assimilative integration: Short-term dynamic psychotherapy for treating affect phobias. *Clinical Psychology: Science and Practice, 8,* 82–97.

McCullough-Vaillant, L. (1997). *Changing Character.* New York: Basic Books.

Miller, S. J., & Binder, J. L. (2002). The effects of manual-based training on treatment fidelity and outcome: A review of the literature on adult individual psychotherapy. *Psychotherapy: Theory, Research, Practice, Training, 39,* 184–198.

Mitchell, S. A. (1988). *Relational Concepts in Psychoanalysis: An Integration.* Cambridge, MA: Harvard University Press.

Mitchell, S. A., & Black, M. J. (1995). *Freud and Beyond: A History of Modern Psychoanalytic Thought.* New York: Basic Books.

Najavits, L., & Strupp, H. H. (1994). Differences in the effectiveness of psychodynamic therapists: A process–outcome study. *Psychotherapy, 31,* 114–123.

Neimeyer, R. A. (1997a). An invitation to constructivist psychotherapies. In R. A. Neimeyer & M. J. Mahoney (Eds.), *Constructivism in Psychotherapy* (pp. 1–10). Washington, DC: American Psychological Association.

Neimeyer, R. A. (1997b). Constructivist psychotherapies: Features, foundations, and future directions. In R. A. Neimeyer & M. J. Mahoney (Eds.), *Constructivism in Psychotherapy* (pp. 11–38). Washington, DC: American Psychological Association.

Neimeyer, R. A., & Mahoney, M. J. (1995). *Constructivism in Psychotherapy.* Washington, DC: American Psychological Association.

Newman, C. F. (1998). The therapeutic relationship and alliance in short-term cognitive therapy. In J. D. Safran & J. C. Muran (Eds.), *The Therapeutic Alliance in Brief Psychotherapy* (pp. 95–122). Washington, DC: American Psychological Association.

Norcross, J. C. (2001). Purposes, processes, and products of the task force on empirically supported therapist relationships. *Psychotherapy: Theory, Research, Practice, Training, 38,* 345–356.

Norcross, J. C. (Ed.). (2002). *Psychotherapy Relationships That Work: Therapist Contributions and Responsiveness to Patient Needs.* New York: Oxford University Press.

Norville, R., Sampson, H., & Weiss, J. (1996). Accurate interpretations and brief psychotherapy outcome. *Psychotherapy Research, 6,* 16–29.

Ogrodniczuk, J. S., & Piper, W. E. (1999). Use of transference interpretations in dynamically oriented individual psychotherapy for patients with personality disorders. *Journal of Personality Disorders, 13,* 297–311.

Ogrodniczuk, J. S., Piper, W. E., Joyce, A. S., & McCallum, M. (1999). Transference interpretations in short-term dynamic psychotherapy. *Journal of Nervous and Mental Disease, 187,* 571–578.

O'Malley, S. S., Foley, S. H., Rounsaville, B. J., Watkins, J. T., Sotsky, S. M., Imber, S. D., & Elkin, I. (1988). Therapist competence and patient outcomes in interpersonal psychotherapy of depression. *Journal of Consulting and Clinical Psychology, 56,* 496–501.

Orlinsky, D. E., & Geller, J. D. (1993). Patients' representations of their therapists and therapy: New measures. In N. E. Miller, L. Luborsky, J. P. Barber, J. P. Docherty (Eds.), *Psychodynamic Treatment Research: A Handbook for Clinical Practice* (pp. 423–466). New York: Basic Books.

Orlinsky, D. E., Grawe, K., & Parks, B. K. (1994). Process and outcome in psycho-therapy—noch einmal. In A E. Bergin & S. L. Garfield (Eds.), *Handbook of Psychotherapy and Behavior Change* (4th ed., pp. 270–378). New York: Wiley.

Patel, V. L., & Groen, G. J. (1991). The general and specific nature of medical expertise: A critical look. In K. A. Ericsson & J. Smith (Eds.), *Toward a General Theory of Expertise* (pp. 93–125). New York: Cambridge University Press.

Patton, M. J. (2000). Counseling psychology training: A matter of good teaching. *The Counseling Psychologist, 28,* 701–711.

Peterfreund, E. (1983). *The Process of Psychoanalytic Therapy: Models and Strategies.* Hillsdale, NJ: Erlbaum.

Piaget, J. (1967). *Six Psychological Studies* (A. Tenzer, Trans.; D. Elkind, Ed.). New York: Random House.

Pine, F. (1990). *Drive, Ego, Object, and Self: A Synthesis for Clinical Work.* New York: Basic Books.

Piper, W. E., & Duncan, S. C. (1999). Object relations theory and short-term dynamic psychotherapy: Findings from the Quality of Object Relations Scale. *Clinical Psychology Review, 19,* 669–685.

Piper, W. E., Joyce, A. S., McCallum, M., & Azim, H. F. (1993). Concentration and correspondence of transference interpretations in short-term psychotherapy. *Journal of Consulting and Clinical Psychology, 61,* 586–595.

Piper, W. E., Joyce, A. A., McCallum, M., & Azim, H. F. (1998). Interpretive and supportive forms of psychotherapy and patient personality variables. *Journal of Consulting and Clinical Psychology, 66,* 558–567.

Piper, W. E., Joyce, A. S., McCallum, M., Azim, H. F., & Ogrodniczuk, J. S. (2002). *Interpretive and Supportive Psychotherapies: Matching Therapy and Patient Personality.* Washington, DC: American Psychological Association.

Piper, W. E., Ogrodniczuk, J. S., Joyce, A. S., McCallum, M., Rosie, J. S., O'Kelly, J. G., & Steinberg, P. I. (1999). Prediction of dropping out in time-limited, interpretive individual psychotherapy. *Psychotherapy, 36,* 114–122.

Polanyi, M. (1967). *The Tacit Dimension.* New York: Doubleday.

Quintana, S. M. (1993). Toward an expanded and updated conceptualization of termination: Implications for short-term individual psychotherapy. *Professional Psychology: Research and Practice, 24,* 426–432.

Quintana, S. M., & Holahan, W. (1992). Termination in short-term counseling: Comparison of successful and unsuccessful cases. *Journal of Counseling Psychology, 39,* 299–305.

Recihelt, S., & Skjerva, J. (2002). Correspondence between supervisors and trainees in their perceptions of supervision events. *Journal of Clinical Psychology, 58,* 759–772.

Reynold, S., Stiles, W. B., Barkham, M., Shapiro, D. A., Hardy, G. E., & Reeves, A. (1996). Acceleration of changes in session impact during contrasting time-limited psychotherapies. *Journal of Consulting and Clinical Psychology, 64,* 577–586.

Safran, J. D., & Segal, Z. V. (1990). *Interpersonal Process in Cognitive Therapy.* New York: Basic Books.

Safran, J. D., & Muran, J. C. (Eds.). (1998). *The Therapeutic Alliance in Brief Psychotherapy.* Washington, DC: American Psychological Association.

Safran, J. D., & Muran, J. C. (2000). *Negotiating the Therapeutic Alliance: A Relational Treatment Guide*. New York: Guilford Press.

Sandifer, M. G., Hordern, A., & Green, L. M. (1970). The psychiatric interview: The impact of the first three minutes. *American Journal of Psychiatry, 126,* 968–973.

Sandler, J., & Sandler, A. M. (1978). On the development of object relationships and affects. *International Journal of Psychoanalysis, 59,* 285–296.

Santayana, G. (1905). *The Life of Reason in Common Sense* (Vol. I). New York: Dover.

Schacht, T. E., Binder, J. L., & Strupp, H. H. (1984). The dynamic focus. In H. H. Strupp & J. L. Binder (Eds.), *Psychotherapy in a New Key: A Guide to Time-Limited Dynamic Psychotherapy* (pp. 65–109). New York: Basic Books.

Schaffer, N. D. (1982). Multidimensional measures of therapist behavior as predictors of outcome. *Psychological Bulletin, 92,* 670–681.

Schaffer, N. D. (1983). Methodological issues of measuring the skillfulness of therapeutic techniques. *Psychotherapy, 20,* 486–493.

Schlesinger, N., & Robbins, F. (1983). *A Developmental View of the Psychoanalytic Process.* New York: International Universities Press.

Schon, D. A. (1983). *The Reflective Practitioner.* New York: Basic Books.

Schon, D. A. (1987). *Educating the Reflective Practitioner.* San Francisco: Jossey-Bass.

Seligman, M. E. P. (1998). *Learned Optimism.* New York: Pocket Books.

Seruya, B. B. (1997). *Empathic Brief Psychotherapy.* Northvale, NJ: Aronson.

Shefler, G., & Tishby, O. (1998). Interjudge reliability and agreement about the patient's central issue in time-limited psychotherapy (TLP) and its relation to TLP outcome. *Psychotherapy Research, 8,* 426–438.

Sifneos, P. E. (1979). *Short-Term Dynamic Psychotherapy.* New York: Plenum Press.

Silberschatz, G., Fretter, P. B., & Curtis, J. T. (1986). How do interpretations influence the process of psychotherapy? *Journal of Consulting and Clinical Psychology, 54,* 646–652.

Spence, D. P. (1982). *Narrative Truth and Historical Truth: Meaning and Interpretation in Psychoanalysis.* New York: Norton.

Stadter, M. (1996). *Object Relations Brief Therapy.* Northvale, NJ: Aronson.

Stern, D. N. (1985). *The Interpersonal World of the Infant.* New York: Basic Books.

Sternberg, R. J. (1977). Component processes in analogic reasoning. *Psychological Review, 84,* 353–378.

Sternberg, R. J., & Horvath, J. A. (Eds.). (1999). *Tacit Knowledge in Professional Practice: Researcher and Practitioner Perspectives.* Mahwah, NJ: Erlbaum.

Strupp, H. H. (1993). The Vanderbilt Psychotherapy Studies: Synopsis. *Journal of Consulting and Clinical Psychology, 61,* 431–433.

Strupp, H. H., & Anderson, T. (1997). On the limitations of therapy manuals. *Clinical Psychology: Science and Practice, 4,* 76–82.

Strupp, H. H., & Binder, J. L. (1984). *Psychotherapy in a New Key: A Guide to Time-Limited Dynamic Psychotherapy.* New York: Basic Books.

Strupp, H. H., Butler, S. F., & Rosser, C. L. (1988). Training in psychodynamic therapy. *Journal of Consulting and Clinical Psychology, 56,* 689–695.

Suh, C. S., O'Malley, S. S., & Strupp, H. H. (1986). The Vanderbilt Process Measures: The Psychotherapy Process Scale (VPSS) and the Negative Indicators

Scale (VNIS). In L. S. Greenberg & W. M. Pinsof (Eds.), *The Psychotherapeutic Process: A Research Handbook* (pp. 285–324). New York: Guilford Press.

Sullivan, H. S. (1954). *The Psychiatric Interview.* New York: Norton.

Ticho, E. (1972). Termination of psychoanalysis: Treatment goals, life goals. *Psychoanalytic Quarterly, 41,* 315–333.

Urist, J. (2000). On the object relational texture of affects. *Journal of Personality Assessment, 75,* 9–17.

Wachtel, P. L. (1993). *Therapeutic Communication: Principles and Effective Practice.* New York: Guilford Press.

Wachtel, P. L. (2002). Termination of therapy: An effort at integration. *Journal of Psychotherapy Integration, 12,* 373–383.

Wachtel, P. L. (2003). The surface and the depths: The metaphor of depth in psychoanalysis and the ways it can mislead. *Contemporary Psychoanalysis, 39,* 5–26.

Wallerstein, R. S. (1989). The psychotherapy research project of the Menninger Foundation: An overview. *Journal of Consulting and Clinical Psychology, 57,* 195–205.

Weston, D. (1988). Transference and information processing. *Clinical Psychology Review, 8,* 161–179.

Whipple, J. L., Lambert, M. J., Vermeerch, D. A., Smart, D. W., Nielsen, S. L., & Hawkings, E. J. (2003). Improving the effects of psychotherapy: The use of early identification of treatment failure and problem-solving strategies in routine practice. *Journal of Counseling Psychology, 50,* 59–68.

Widiger, T. A. (1997). Mental disorders as discrete clinical conditions. Dimensional versus categorical classifications. In S. M. Turner & M. Hersen (Eds.), *Adult Psychopathology and Diagnosis* (3rd ed., pp. 3–23). New York: Wiley.

Wiley, D. B. (1984). Kohut, Kernberg, and accusatory interpretations. *Psychotherapy, 21,* 353–364.

Winnicott, D. W. (1971). *Playing and Reality.* New York: Basic Books.

Wiser, S., & Arnow, B. (2001). Emotional experiencing: To facilitate or regulate? *Journal of Clinical Psychology: In Session, 57,* 157–168.

Wolberg, L. (1980). *Handbook of Short-Term Psychotherapy.* New York: Grune & Stratton.

Zois, C. L., & Scarpa, M. (1997). *Short-Term Therapy Techniques.* Northvale, NJ: Aronson.

Index